THE FRAGRANT
FLOWER GARDEN

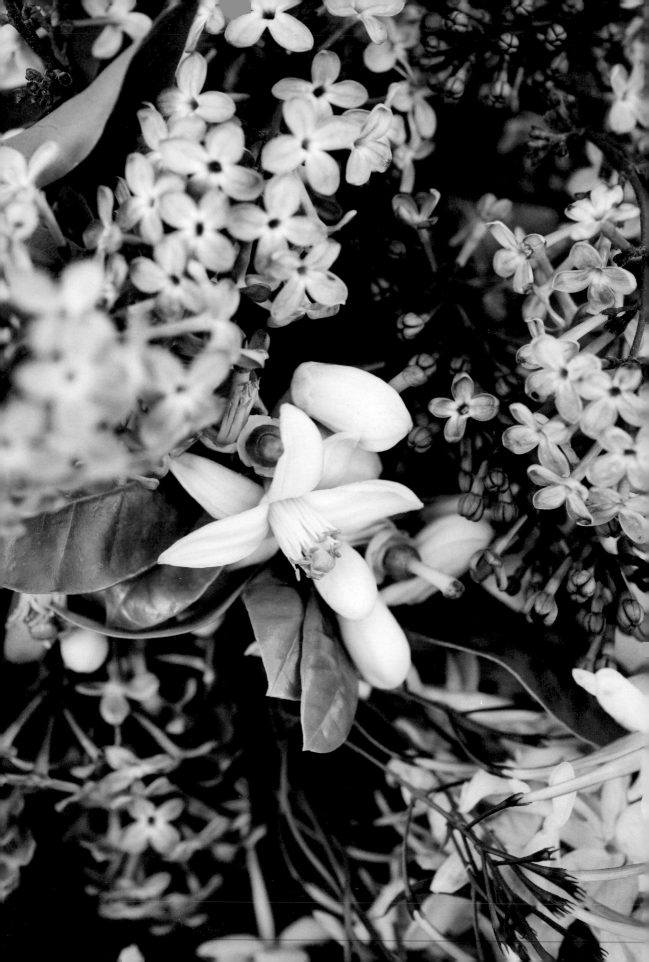

THE FRAGRANT FLOWER GARDEN

Growing, Arranging & Preserving Natural Scents

STEFANI BITTNER & ALETHEA HARAMPOLIS

PHOTOGRAPHS BY DAVID FENTON

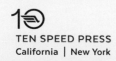

TEN SPEED PRESS
California | New York

CONTENTS

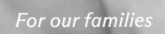

For our families

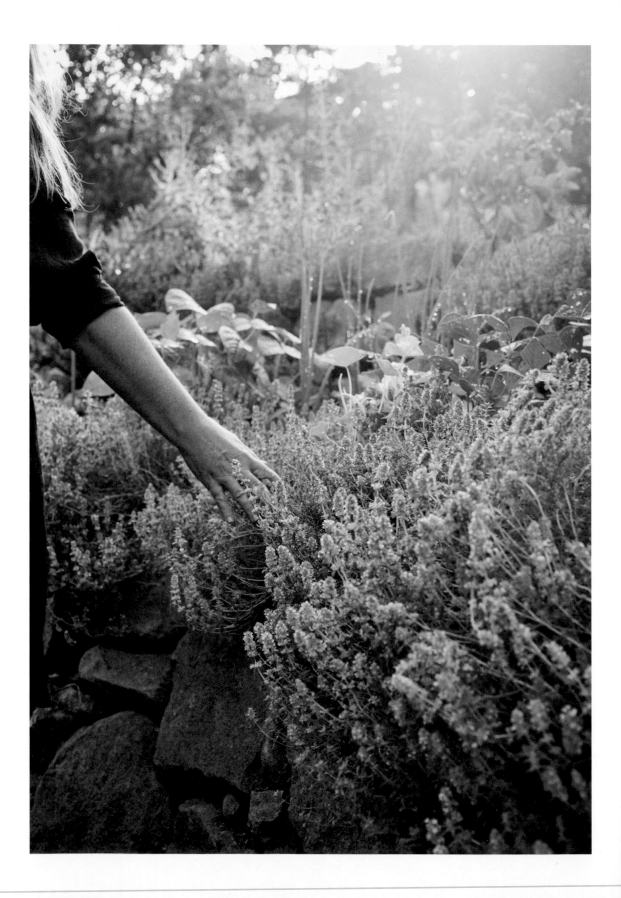

INTRODUCTION

A garden can benefit and enrich your life in so many unexpected ways. As an extension of your living space, a garden can be a quiet place to relax with a book or a place to gather and celebrate with friends. A garden can do more than just look pretty. It can be a place of solace, joy, beauty, and rejuvenation. Including scented plants in your garden creates a sense of magic and wonder, as their fragrances evoke memories, lift your spirits, soothe your nerves, surprise and delight visitors, and elevate your garden to a place of heavenly bliss.

If you are passionate about gardening, you know that it is a labor of love, and you know that the time and energy you put into gardening will reward you in many ways. Creating and maintaining a fragrant garden requires no more time or effort than that of any other garden, but the bounty and blessings are multiplied, resulting in a landscape that is both beautiful and wondrously fragrant. When you bring your flower harvests indoors, you are further rewarded with fragrance and beauty inside your home.

Chapters one and two explore the world of scented plants that can enhance both your garden and your home. You can experience one of the greatest joys of a fragrant flower garden by bringing the flowers' intoxicating scents indoors. Whether you're creating gorgeous floral arrangements or making all-natural beauty products, fragrant plants can enhance your life and embellish your living space in many ways. In chapters three and four, you'll learn about ways to use your scented bounty to enrich your home through garden-grown arrangements, herbal hydrosol, natural perfumes, flower tinctures, potpourri, and so much more.

One of the added benefits of creating beauty products from the garden is that they are healthy, both for the environment and for your body. Many commercially available scented products and perfumes are created from synthetic chemicals. You can create homemade perfumes and scented beauty and home products directly from the natural raw materials growing in your own garden, without the chemicals!

HOW TO USE THIS BOOK

This book includes many plants that can be grown in all USDA hardiness zones (see page 37), but it is not a fragrant plant encyclopedia. The goal of this book is to help you learn about how to grow and engage with fragrance and then seek out more plants that grow in your region to include in your garden.

One of the best places to start is at your local botanical garden or independent plant nursery, where you can talk to knowledgeable staff about fragrant plants. You can also get to know the fragrant plants that flourish in your part of the world by taking time to "stop and smell the roses." As you encounter a fragrant flower in a garden or nursery, lean over the flower, cup your hands around your nose and mouth, and inhale. To experience a plant's fragrant foliage, reach out and gently rub the plant's leaf. Doing this will release the plant's scent into the air and probably onto your hand.

It's hard to describe scent. Adjectives are often used that tell you nothing about what a plant smells like. Words like "lovely," "pleasant," "scented," and "intoxicating" tell you nothing except that a plant is, well, lovely. In this book, we make comparisons to familiar scents to describe a plant's fragrance. For example, *Sarcococca* (sweet box) smells like vanilla (which is lovely in the winter when it blooms). But sometimes the descriptive word is simply the plant's name. For us, rosemary smells like rosemary. It is a highlight of our California winter gardens when the plant is in bloom, and it's the backdrop of the hot summer days when we tend to the garden daily. Rosemary's scent is consistent and grounding. But that does not tell you what the plant smells like, but rather the emotional experience attached to the scent. Keep in mind that scent is subjective, emotive, and personal. It's okay if you do not agree with our description of a plant's fragrance, but we hope that you agree that these plants are worth seeking out and including in your garden space.

The gardens shared in this book are designed, installed, and maintained by Stefani's company, Homestead Design Collective. The folks in the garden photos included here are not models, but part of our garden community at Homestead and our families. They are real gardeners in the real gardens that we have created. Many of the beautiful arrangements and all of the beauty products in the book were created by Alethea, who owns Studio Choo, a boutique floral design studio. She is the coauthor (with Jill Rizzo) of *The Flower Recipe Book* and *The Wreath Recipe Book*, and she is a perfumer. Also included are arrangements created by our friend Juliette Surnamer, a Los Angeles–based florist. We have been so lucky to work with photographer David Fenton on this book and both of Stefani's other books (*The Beautiful Edible Garden* and *Harvest*). In this book, David's photography beautifully captures the emotive experience of the fragrant flower garden.

A garden can be a constant source of aromatic inspiration, both indoors and out. The good news is that all it takes is getting to know fragrant flowers and plants and incorporating them in your garden. We hope you enjoy the journey of transforming your garden into one of both beauty and enchanting fragrance. We are excited to share our expertise in gardening, floristry, and perfumery with you.

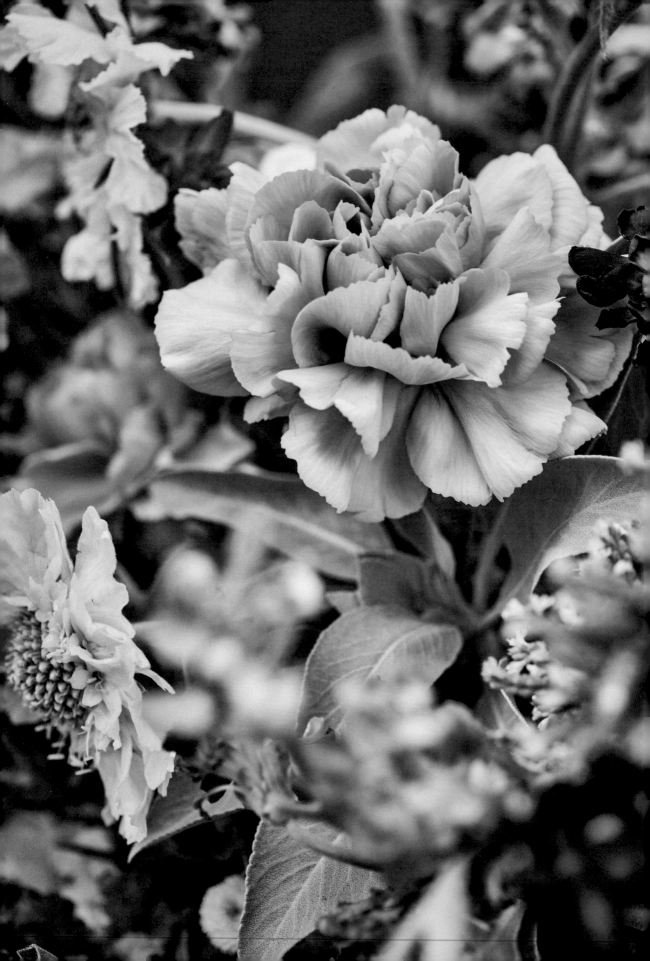

CHAPTER ONE

GARDENING WITH FRAGRANCE

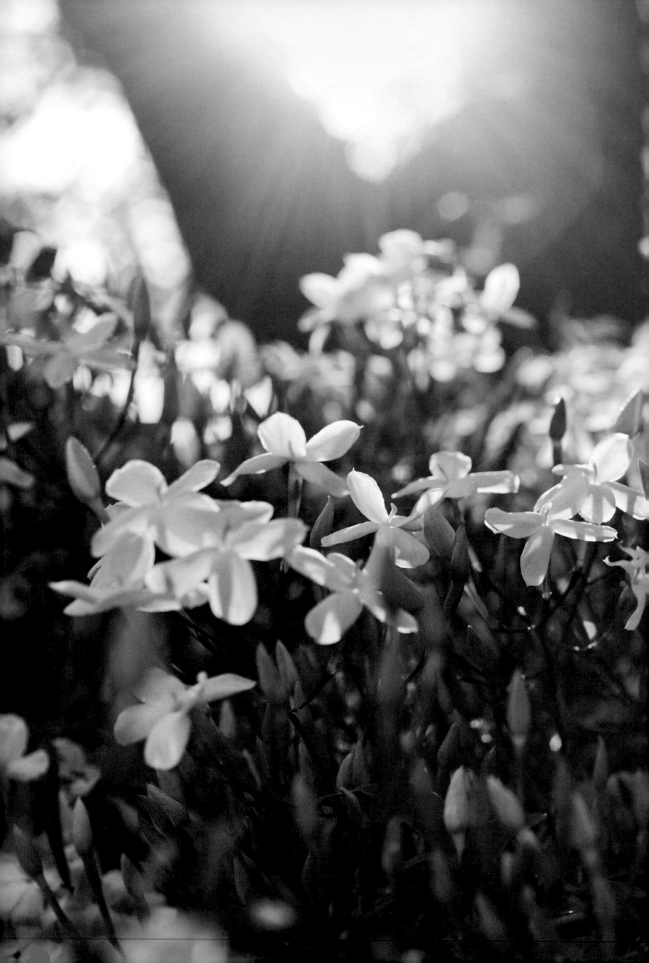

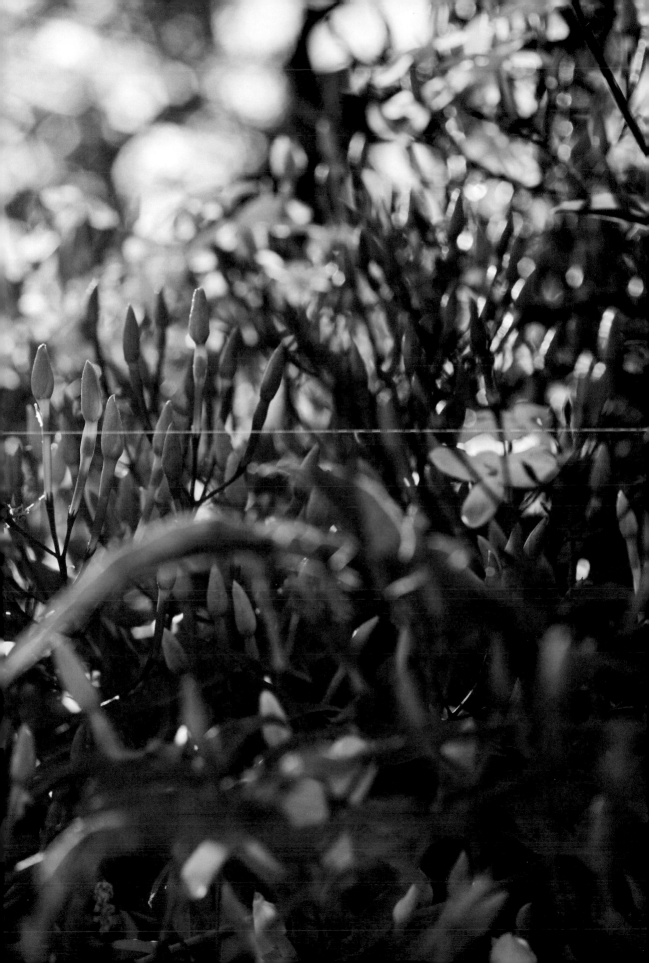

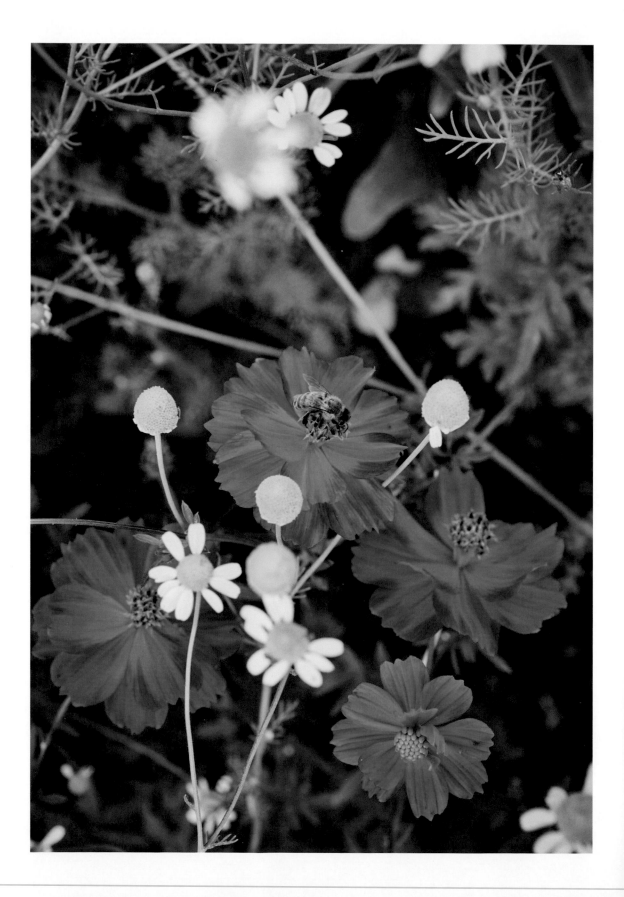

Scent can have a powerful connection to memory. Fragrant gardens tell stories and hold the memories of those who live with them, and choosing particular scented plants for your garden can honor these memories and help you create new ones. Fragrance helps you explore and experience the garden and is an integral part of the garden experience and an important design consideration when planning a garden space. This chapter provides some basic gardening requirements to get you off on the right foot for making a successful fragrant garden. It also shares some garden design techniques to help you make the most of the fragrant plants in your garden.

chamomile,
'Sulphur' cosmo
with bee

LET'S TALK ABOUT PLANT SEX

Planting a diverse fragrant garden is one of the easiest ways we can help support local pollinators. Flowers developed their fragrances not for us, but for their pollinators. A flower's scent is a signal that it is ready to be pollinated. Pollen is basically plant sperm, and it's required by flowering plants in order to reproduce. Yes, pollination is simply about plant sex, and fragrance is nature's signal that plants are ready for it. A flower includes the plant's sexual parts that are used in reproduction. After the pollen fertilizes the flower, the plant produces fruits or seeds.

Pollinators are often insects such as bees and butterflies or animals such as hummingbirds, but wind can also distribute pollen. Often, pollinators (and people) can smell a flower long before they see it. The time of day when a flower releases its scent tells you a lot about who pollinates that flower. Flowers that are most fragrant during the day are typically pollinated by butterflies, hummingbirds, and bees. Night-fragrant flowers are typically pollinated by moths and bats. Some flowers release very specific scents to attract very specific pollinators. For example, many unpleasant or foul-smelling flowers attract particular beetles and flies that they require for pollination. These different flowering times and scents decrease competition among plants for their pollinator partners. The plant reproduction system is really quite amazing.

GROWING CONDITIONS—SOIL, SUN, WATER

Like all plants, each fragrant plant has specific needs with regard to soil, light, and water conditions. Before you begin designing and planting, make sure that you know what conditions exist in your garden space, so that you can group plants by their specific soil, light, and water needs.

All living things need water, food, and air to survive, and plants get all three from the soil. Healthy soil is a determining factor in whether a garden is lush and beautiful or struggling. The most important investment you can make in your garden is to include healthy soil. Organic compost is the answer to most gardens' soil needs. If a garden has sandy or clay soil, adding organic compost will help the soil reach the more desired loamy state—loamy soil is fluffy, fertile soil that plant roots love. It's great if you are able to make your own compost, but most garden compost bins are not large enough to create compost for an entire garden. Luckily, most garden centers carry organic compost and soil products.

THE BENEFITS OF ORGANIC GARDENING

Many folks buy organic vegetables and fruit, flowers, and beauty products to avoid bringing pesticides and other toxins into their homes. When growing plants to harvest for food or for making perfumes or other fragrant skin products, you should keep a few principles in mind. Just as you want to avoid ingesting toxins and pesticides in garden-grown food, you should avoid applying toxins and pesticides to your skin, where it can be absorbed into the body. Before using any part of a plant for consumption, make sure that it has not been sprayed with chemicals or pesticides. Consider roses, for example. Many people don't realize that all roses produce edible petals that can be used in the kitchen or used to make natural scented products. But the way you treat and grow the rose plant determines whether or not the petals are safe to use. This is easy to do if you grow your own roses or other fragrant flowers. If you have not transitioned your garden to organic care, this is a good time to start.

Plants need light to grow. That's why, before you start planting, it's important to identify how much sunlight each area receives. Gardens often include areas with several different levels of sun exposure. Go outside at midday and take a look at your garden space. The south-facing parts of your garden will typically receive full sun for six to ten hours per day if there are no trees or large structures that cast shade in those areas. Unshaded, west-facing parts of your garden will typically receive sunlight from midday until sundown, a good five to eight hours, depending on the time of year. This is also considered full sun conditions. An unshaded, east-facing area in your garden will receive approximately three to five hours of sunlight per day, which is considered part sun or part shade. Lastly, the north-facing parts of your garden may be in shade throughout the day if they do not receive direct sunlight. This is full shade.

Plants require different amounts of light. Nurseries often include tags in plant pots that list their sun exposure needs—full sun, part sun, part shade, or full shade. Before you set out a plant, make sure that you know the plant's light needs and the type of light provided in each area of your garden. You'll find light requirements listed for the fragrant plants featured in this book on pages 41–142. A plant that grows best in the shade should be planted in a shady spot, not in a full sun area, where it will not thrive. And by the same token, a plant that requires full sun will not thrive if it's planted in a shady area.

It's also important to understand your garden's water needs. How much water your garden requires is determined by the plants you choose and by your location. Do you live in a Mediterranean climate with dry summers? Or are you gardening in an area with wet summers? A plant that needs a lot of water to thrive isn't a good choice for a garden in an arid environment. Likewise, a plant that thrives with low amounts of summer water may not be happy in a garden that receives lots of summer rain. To determine a plant's water requirements, check the nursery tag or search online. If you are unsure of your climate, you can learn a lot by determining your garden's hardiness zone (see page 207).

Even if your area is not affected by drought, an efficient watering system is one of the most important investments you can make. A watering or irrigation system should be able to direct different amounts of water to different sections of your garden according to the amount of sunlight received and the plants' particular needs. To make the most of an irrigation system and provide an appropriate amount of water for your plants, group plants with similar water requirements together so that they can be included in the same water station or irrigation line. Plants with similar water needs will thrive.

SEASONAL & HOURLY SCENTS

Each flowering plant has a blooming season. Within each general blooming season—spring, summer, fall, and winter—are early-, middle-, and late-season bloomers. For continuous fragrance in the garden and to avoid an abundance of flowers and fragrances occurring at the same time, choose plants with staggered blooming times. A fragrant garden should evolve and change throughout the blooming season.

A single type of plant may include specific varieties or cultivars that bloom early, middle, or late in the season. Consider lilacs, for example. 'Declaration' lilac (*Syringa × hyacinthiflora* 'Declaration') blooms in early spring for a glorious few weeks. Later, midseason lilac cultivar *S. vulgaris* 'Charles Joly' displays its magenta flowers. In late spring, the flowers of *S. vulgaris* 'Ludwig Spaeth' erupt in bloom. If you plant all three in your garden, instead of enjoying just two or three weeks of lilac blooms, you'll have more than six weeks to enjoy fragrant lilac flowers. If lilacs are a favorite and you have the space to include three or more shrubs in your garden, why not diversify within the plant species and lengthen the fragrant lilac season?

Fragrance in the garden also changes with the time of day. Some flowers, including roses, are at their most fragrant in the morning hours, some fragrant flowers peak in the high heat of the afternoon, and others are best early in the evening. There are even some night-blooming flowers (see page 19) to enjoy. Getting to know bloom times, whether hourly or seasonal, will help you design your garden space for continual fragrance.

Combining Fragrant Plants in the Landscape

A fragrant garden should include both heady (strong) and subtle scents. Some flower scents pack a wallop, like the exuberant burst of spring-blooming lilacs. Others produce more subtle fragrances and require patience and up-close interactions, such as calendula flowers, which smell like hay. Like all things in life, fragrant gardens tend to be most successful when they are balanced. A good combination of both heady and subtle scents combined with seasonal scents planted in succession will keep you returning to the garden for more.

You can think of subtly scented flowers and plants as the foundations of the fragrant garden. They can be long-lasting, steady fragrance providers—garden elders that are consistent, but not flashy. Fragrant foliage is generally more subtle than scented flowers and the fragrance lasts throughout the growing season.

On the other hand, short-lived, abundantly fragrant plants are the rock stars of the garden. Blooming flowers often produce a brief, but glorious, experience that is all-encompassing. They garner attention, and everyone wants to bask in their fragrance when they are in the spotlight. When flowers are in bloom, you can harvest frequently and fill your vases to capture and preserve their scent.

Keep the strength of the plant's fragrance in mind as you determine where you will place it in the garden. If a flower's scent can be detected throughout the garden, for example, the plant does not need to be front and center for you to enjoy its fragrance. Likewise, if a plant's scent is activated by touch or is so subtle that you need to be up close to appreciate it, you can place it near a pathway, where you can enjoy the fragrance along the way. You can also think about fragrant plants' bloom time when planning your garden. Within a planting, for example, you can combine heady, strongly scented flowering shrubs with plants of differing bloom times. Each plant can then have its fabulous fragrant moment in the garden, and the heady scents of particular flowers and plants will permeate the garden.

As you fill your space, avoid planting different strongly scented, simultaneously blooming plants adjacent to one another to ensure that each plant's unique fragrance can be experienced individually. Suppose, for example, that you want to include two night-blooming, strongly fragrant plants such as angel's trumpets (*Brugmansia* spp.) and night-blooming jasmine (*Cestrum nocturnum*) in your garden. The bloom times of both plants overlap in the summer, so planting them on opposite sides of the garden will make the most of their unique scents.

Here are a few favorite fragrant plant combination ideas:

Full sun, low-water shrubs and perennials

These waterwise plants release fragrance when you brush up against them. None of their scents is strong enough to overpower the others. Instead, each plant invites passersby to explore the garden.

Breath of heaven: *Coleonema* spp.

Ironwort: *Sideritis* spp.

Lavender: *Lavandula* spp.

Rosemary: *Rosmarinus officinalis*

Sage: Cleveland sage (*Salvia clevelandii*), white sage (*S. apiana*)

Part and full shade shrubs with successive bloom times

Butterfly ginger flowers in summer, and the flowering shrubs take turns blooming: osmanthus in early winter, sweet box in midwinter. Their scents will not compete because their blooming periods are staggered. Plant the following shrubs under the Champok tree's canopy.

Butterfly ginger: *Hedychium coronarium*

Mexican orange: *Choisya ternata*

Sweet box: *Sarcococca* spp.

Sweet osmanthus: *Osmanthus fragrans*

Winter daphne: *Daphne odora*

Fenceline shrubs and perennials

Plant early spring–blooming lilacs, late spring/early summer–blooming mock orange, and summer-blooming butterfly bush along a fence. As one shrub finishes flowering, another begins. Climbing roses can be trained along the fence. The scent of almond verbena complements the sweeter floral fragrance of the summer-blooming roses and butterfly bush.

Butterfly bush: *Buddleia* spp.

Climbing roses

Lilacs: *Syringa* spp.

Mock orange: *Philadelphus* spp.

Sweet almond verbena: *Aloysia virgata*

Full sun rose bed planting

These three make excellent companion plants. The growing requirements and overall size of calamint and dwarf lavender complement those of roses, and they offer fragrant substitutes for catmint (*Nepeta* spp.)—a classic rose companion plant. The fragrant flowering perennials fill the lower part of the planting bed, covering the bare and often thorny stems of the roses.

Calamint: *Calamintha* spp.

Dwarf lavenders

Roses

Tea-lover's garden

The herbaceous fragrances of these tea-garden plants blend well together—in the garden and in a cup of tea. All have the same growing requirements and are happy to comingle in the same planting bed or container.

Anise hyssop: *Agastache foeniculum*

'Berggarten' sage: *Salvia officinalis* 'Berggarten'

German chamomile: *Matricaria chamomilla*

Lemon balm: *Melissa officinalis*

Lemon bee balm: *Monarda citriodora*

Lemon verbena: *Aloysia citrodora*

Mint: *Mentha sp.*

'Tangerine' sage: *Salvia elegans* 'Tangerine'

Tulsi basil: *Ocimum tenuifolium*

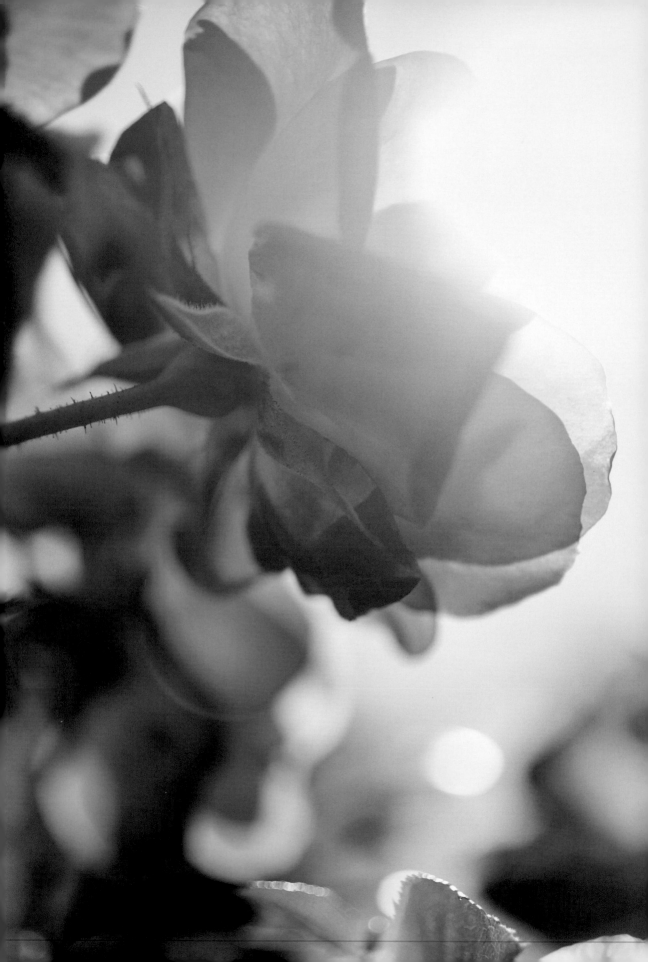

FOCAL POINTS & DESTINATIONS

Many permanent elements can serve as focal points and/or destinations in front- and backyard gardens, including gathering spaces, a garden bench, or a water feature. A dedicated vegetable and cut flower garden or a special tree can also be a focal point. You can emphasize special elements by designing pathways that lead to them. A circular path in a back garden, for example, can be designed to lead to multiple destinations. Placing focal points at a distance, rather than directly outside your back door, can lengthen a view and make a small backyard seem larger. When choosing a fragrant plant as a focal point or destination, make sure that it is a long-lived, an evergreen, or a sculptural plant (if winter-dormant).

Favorite fragrant focal point/destination trees, shrubs, and perennials

Angel's trumpets: *Brugmansia* spp.

Citrus

Frangipani: *Plumeria* spp.

Olive: *Olea europaea*

'Joseph's Coat' rose

Roses

PERENNIAL AND ANNUAL PLANTS

It is important to understand the lifespan of a plant before you choose a location for it. Perennial plants, which usually live longer than two years, are the anchors in the garden that provide structure, screening, and focal points. These plants grow with us as gardeners. Annual plants typically live for a single year or growing season. They have a peak flowering season that is glorious and then they are done. These are not good plants to use as anchors in the garden or landscape because of their ephemeral nature; instead, they are celebrated for their fabulous flowers. Sprinkle annuals among perennial plantings, typically at the front of the beds as seasonal accents, or grow them in dedicated annual beds (see page 23).

ANCHOR PLANTS IN THE LANDSCAPE

Along with permanent elements, anchor plants help create the garden's structural framework. Even in winter, when deciduous plants lose their leaves, your garden can include strong elements that provide visual interest. In warmer climates, anchor plants are ideally evergreen, and in colder climates, where more plants are deciduous, an ideal anchor plant should provide vertical interest or an interesting branch structure. Following are a few of our favorite fragrant anchor plants to use for hedging and for screening to hide unwanted site lines.

Favorite fragrant anchor plants for hedging and screening

Bay laurel: *Laurus nobilis*

Camellia 'High Fragrance'

Champak: *Magnolia champaca*

False holly: *Osmanthus heterophyllus*

Lavender: *Lavandula* spp.

Mexican orange: *Choisya ternata*

Rosemary: *Rosmarinus officinalis*

Sweet osmanthus: *Osmanthus fragrans*

Favorite fragrant anchor vines and climbers for fences and arbors

Climbing roses

Honeysuckle: *Lonicera* spp.

Jasmine: *Jasminum* spp.

Passion flower: *Passiflora* spp.

Wisteria

NIGHT-FRAGRANT PLANTS

Night-blooming fragrant plants typically begin releasing their scents in the late afternoon or evening, often continuing until morning. Use these plants in areas where you like to gather in the evening, such as a terrace or patio, hot tub, or fire pit. Summer night bloomers are wonderful additions near or beneath a bedroom window; open the window to enjoy their fragrance. Plant them near landscape light fixtures along a garden path so that you can see them as well as enjoy their fragrance.

Favorite night-blooming plants

Angel's trumpets: *Brugmansia* spp.

Flowering tobacco: *Nicotiana* spp.

Night-blooming jasmine: *Cestrum nocturnum*

Night phlox: *Zaluzianskya capensis*

Night-scented stock: *Matthiola bicornis*

Phlox: *Phlox drummondii*

Pinks: *Dianthus* spp.

Regal lily: *Lilium regale*

Star jasmine: *Trachelospermum jasminoides*

Wisteria

GROUND COVERS & LOW-GROWING PLANTS

Don't overlook the smallest plants in the garden! Using ground covers and low-growing plants in and around pathways can have an impactful effect in the fragrant garden. Repeated plantings of ground covers can establish a balanced and cohesive look and provide a place for a fragrant stroll in the garden.

Favorite fragrant ground covers

'Berggarten' sage: *Salvia officinalis* 'Berggarten'

Calamint: *Calamintha* spp.

Corsican mint: *Mentha requienii*

Creeping thyme: *Thymus serpyllum*

'Dwarf Greek' oregano: *Origanum* spp.

'Elfin' thyme: *Thymus serpyllum* 'Elfin'

Ironwort: *Sideritis cypria*

Lavenders: *Lavandula* × *intermedia* 'Edelweiss', *L. angustifolia* 'Munstead'

Roman chamomile: *Chamaemelum nobile*

Sweet woodruff: *Galium odoratum*

'White Anniversary' oregano: *Origanum vulgare* 'White Anniversary'

'Pomegranate' yarrow, chocolate cosmos, culinary thyme, 'Elfin' thyme

DON'T EAT WHAT YOU STEP ON

Remember these common-sense safety tips regarding fragrant, low-growing plants in pathways: Don't harvest low-growing plants for eating or making home fragrance. These plants are often trodden upon by soiled shoes and animals, and those that edge driveways or sidewalks may have been used by neighbors' pets. Enjoy these plants for their beauty and fragrance, leaving their blooms for pollinators or harvesting for the vase only.

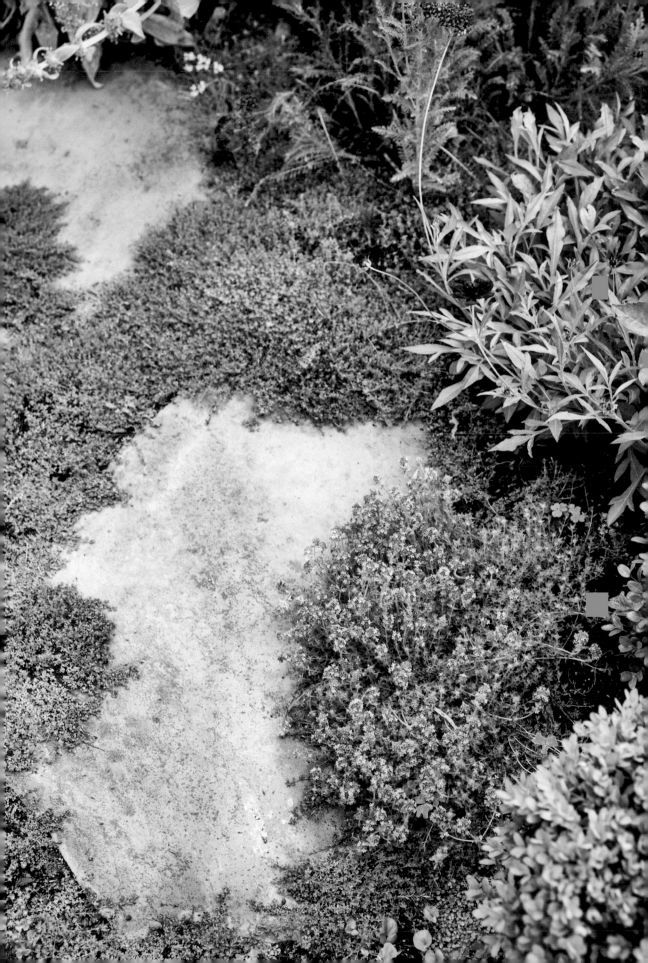

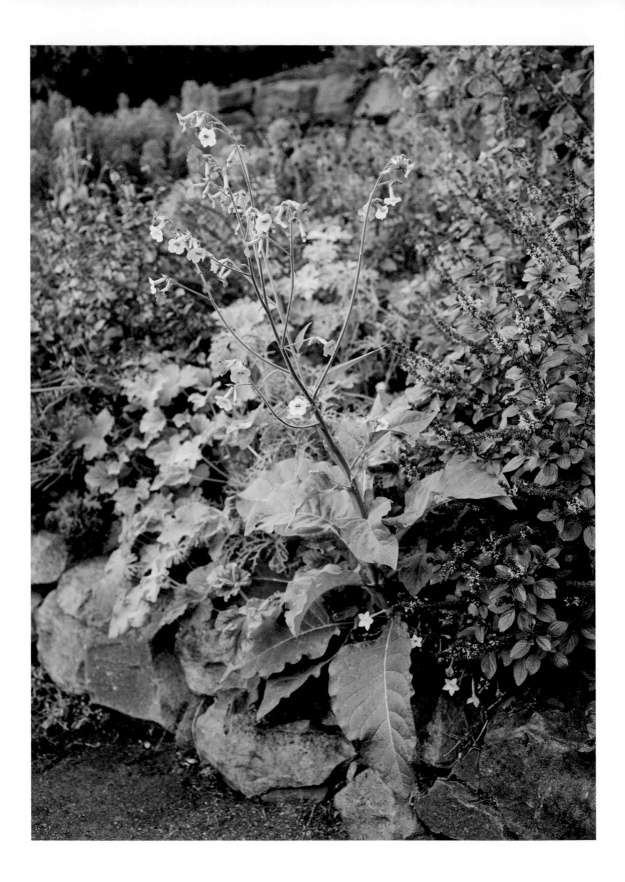

DEDICATED FRAGRANT PLANTING BEDS

Cut Flower Gardens

Annual flowers grown for cutting allow you to have favorite varieties on hand in one place and an opportunity to grow some of the harder-to-find varieties that you admire. If your space allows for multiple dedicated annual beds, we love to take inspiration from the flower arrangement itself when designing cut flower gardens. The three unique parts of an arrangement—focal flowers (the stars that demand attention in a vase), secondary flowers (flowers that provide direction or movement in the vase and are often smaller headed than the focal flowers that help fill out the arrangement with additional color, texture, and fragrance), and filler (also referred to as layered greenery)—are planted in their own separate beds. Planting your dedicated annual beds in these groupings is a great way to make sure that you are growing all of the components for your arrangements. As you explore the dedicated annual beds, you'll compose your arrangement in hand as you harvest groupings from each bed. Aesthetically the characteristics that make the flowers and plants focal, secondary, and filler in arrangements also look good planted together in the individual beds.

Once you have this design in place, you can also explore your greater garden landscape and nearby cut flower garden perennial beds for additional arrangement material. For example, the leaves of your lilac can be an arrangement's foliage filler, or a branch of a lemon tree can be an arrangement's focal. In addition, many focal flowers are perennials and will be grown in the landscape planting beds surrounding the dedicated annual beds. Roses, peonies, irises, and lilacs should not take up valued annual bed space. They will also not appreciate the turnover and disruption to their roots that can happen as annuals come and go. But when it comes to annual flower "crops," the three-bed system is a great way to think about and organize your cut flower garden.

These dedicated beds can be raised beds made of food-safe materials such as redwood, cedar, or quarry stone, or they may be in-ground beds bordered with food-safe materials. To keep the beds from becoming eyesores during the off season, surround them with permanent features, such as

'Chocolate Peppermint' scented geranium, 'Marshmallow' flowering tobacco, 'Mountain Magic' flowering basil

hardscape, fragrant small trees or shrubs, or perennial planting beds. Annual plants in these dedicated beds can live their brief lives without having to carry the aesthetic of the overall garden space.

If you plant your dedicated annual beds with these elements in mind, you can grow all of the components required for every arrangement. In addition, the characteristics that make the flowers and plants focal, secondary, and filler in arrangements will also look aesthetically pleasing in your flower beds.

If your garden has space for fewer dedicated annual beds—or none at all—you can plant annuals in dedicated spaces at the front of your perennial beds. Keep in mind that perennial roots do not appreciate being disturbed by repetitive, short-term annual plantings, so make sure the annuals are planted with plenty of space to avoid this. Containers can also be great for annual plants.

The one place in the garden that we often deviate from a landscape color palette are the dedicated annual cut flower beds. If you want to plant a rainbow of color—this is the place to do it. That being said, if you gravitate toward a particular color palette in your arrangements, you can plant for that specific palette as well. If you're looking for color palette ideas, three color palettes we often recommend are Dusky, Bright, and Silver/White. The Dusky palette includes muted color shades from apricot to rose to burgundy to brown/black. "Bright" is what its name implies—all of the brighter jewel-toned shades. Silver/White provides the contrast of lighter tones.

Following are a few of our favorite perennial and annual cutting flowers in each of these palettes.

'Villandry' marigold, bachelor's button, chamomile, 'African Blue' flowering basil

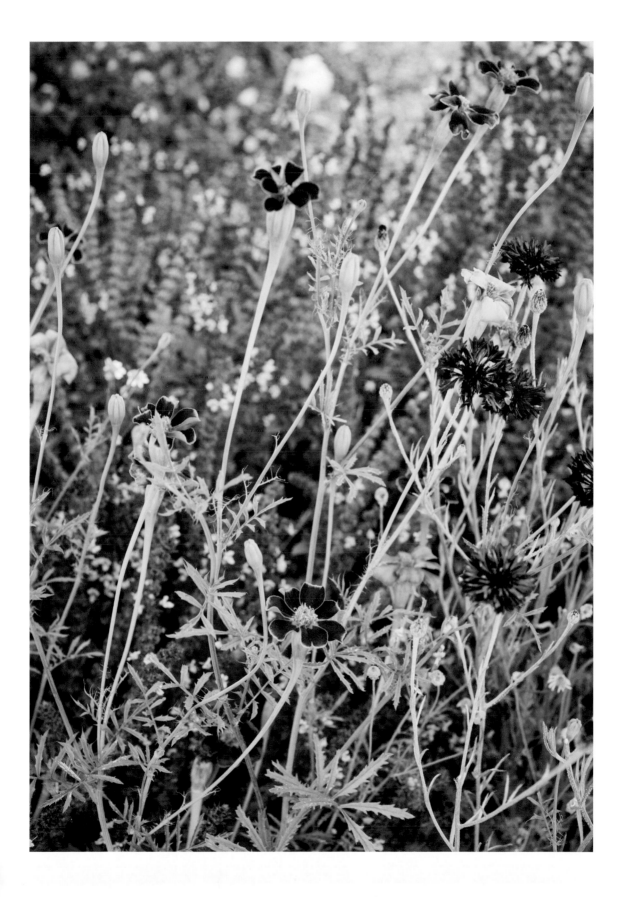

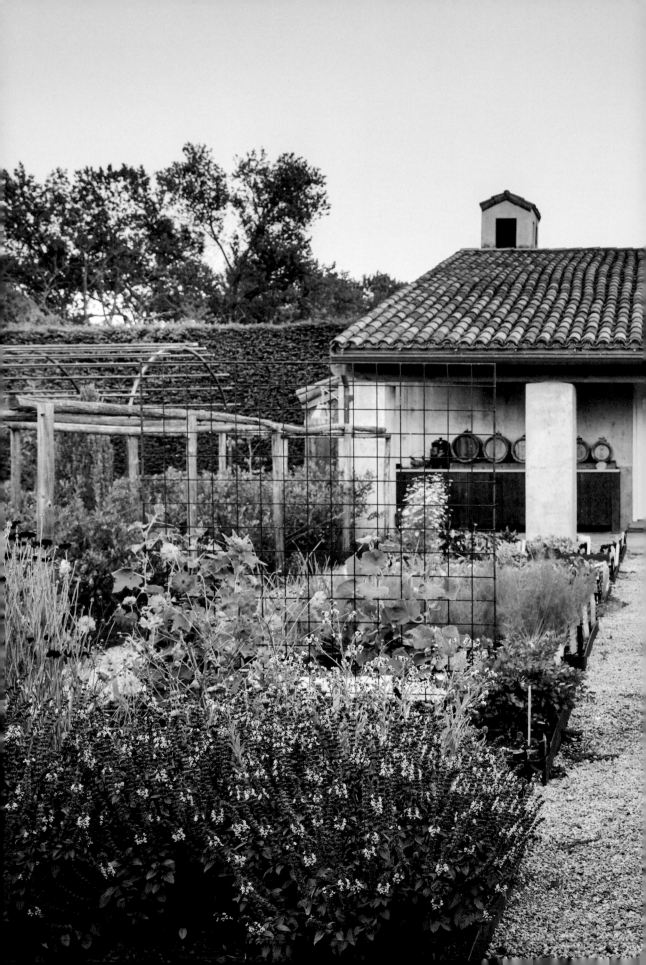

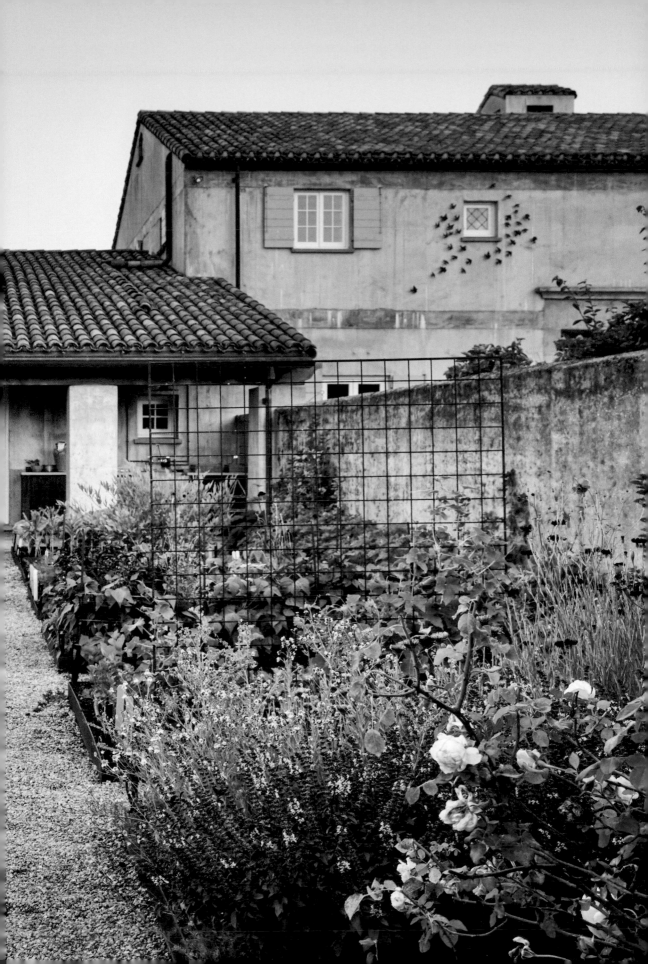

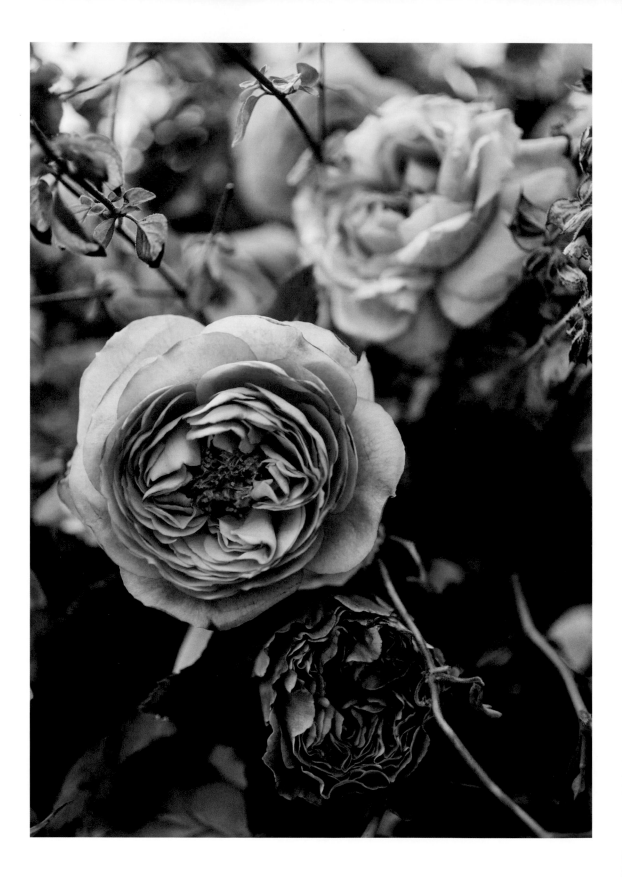

Dusky palette

FOCAL FLOWERS

Bearded irises: *Iris* 'Funday Monday', 'Gingersnap' (smells like root beer!), 'Rum is the Reason'

Lilacs: *Syringa × hyacinthiflora* 'Lavender Lady', *S. vulgaris* 'Sensation'

Lilies: *Lilium* 'Firebolt', 'Nymph', 'Pink Perfection Group'

Peonies: *Paeonia* 'Pink Hawaiian Coral', *P. lactiflora* 'Sarah Bernhardt'

Roses: *Rosa* Abraham Darby ('Auscot'), Emily Brontë ('Ausearnshaw'), Munstead Wood ('Ausbernard')

SECONDARY FLOWERS

Bee balm: *Monarda* 'Raspberry Wine'

Calendula: *Calendula* 'Bronze Beauty'

Chocolate cosmos: *Cosmos atrosanguineus*

Flowering tobaccos: *Nicotiana langsdorffii* 'Bronze Queen', 'Hot Chocolate'

Garden mignonette: *Reseda odorata*

Phlox: *Phlox drummondii* 'Cherry Caramel', 'Crème Brûlée', 'Sugar Stars'

Pinks: *Dianthus barbatus* 'Sooty', *D. chinensis* 'Black Velvet and Lace'

Snapdragon: *Antirrhinum majus* 'Chantilly Light Salmon'

Stock: *Matthiola incana* 'Antique Pink', 'Iron Apricot', 'Iron Rose', 'Vintage Brown'

Sweet peas: *Lathyrus odoratus* 'Castlewellen', 'Nimbus', 'Suzy Zee'

Yarrows: *Achillea millefolium* 'Apricot Delight', 'Summer Pastels', 'Terracotta'

FILLERS

Basil: *Ocimum basilicum* 'Magic Mountain', 'Wild Magic'

Four o'clock: *Mirabilis jalapa* 'Salmon Sunset'

Scented geraniums: *Pelargonium* 'Chocolate Mint', 'Skeleton Rose'

Bright palette

FOCAL FLOWERS

Bearded irises: *Iris* 'Colorista', 'Valentino', 'Ziggy'

Hyacinths: *Hyacinthus orientalis* 'Double Royal Navy', 'Woodstock'

Lilacs: *Syringa × hyacinthiflora* 'Old Glory', *S. vulgaris* 'Yankee Doodle'

Lilies: *Lilium* 'Budapest', 'Golden Splendor Group', 'LeVern Friemann'

Peony: *Paeonia* 'Bartzella'

Roses: *Rosa* Boscobel ('Auscousin'), Double Delight ('Andeli'), Lady of Shalott ('Ausnyson')

SECONDARY FLOWERS

Calendula: *Calendula officinalis* 'Bull's Eye', 'Indian Prince', 'Orange Button'

Freesia: *Freesia* Double Pink

Marigold: *Tagetes* 'Villandry'

Phlox: *Phlox drummondii* 'Grandiflora Starry Eyes Blend'

Pink: *Dianthus* Amazon 'Neon Rose Magic'

Snapdragon: *Antirrhinum majus* 'Sherbet Toned Chantilly Mix'

Sweet peas: *Lathyrus odoratus* 'Blue Shift', 'Carlotta', 'Jacqueline Ann'

Yarrows: *Achillea millefolium* 'Flavorburst Summer Shades', 'Pomegranate'

FILLERS

Basil: *Ocimum* 'African Blue'

Four o'clock: *Mirabilis jalapa* 'Marbles Mix'

Scented geraniums: *Pelargonium* 'Golden Lemon', 'Lemon Meringue', 'Phyllis'

Signet marigolds: *Tagetes tenuifolia* 'Lemon Gem', 'Lemon Star', 'Red Gem', 'Tangerine Gem'

Silver/white palette

FOCAL FLOWERS

Bearded iris: *Iris* 'Immortality'

Lilac: *Syringa* × *hyacinthiflora* 'Angel White'

Lilies: Formosa lily (*Lilium formosanum*), *L.* 'Pink Snowflake'

Stock: *Matthiola incana* 'Buttercream'

Peony: *Paeonia lactiflora* 'Festiva Maxima'

Rose: *Rosa* Desdemona 'Auskindling'

Tuberose: *Agave amica*

SECONDARY FLOWERS

Calendula: *Calendula officinalis* 'Ivory Princess'

Daffodil: *Narcissus* spp.

Flowering tobaccos: *Nicotiana alata* 'Grandiflora', 'Jasmine';
N. × *hybrida* 'Starlight Dancer'

Freesia: *Freesia laxa* var. *alba*

German chamomile: *Matricaria chamomilla*

Heliotrope: *Heliotropium arborescens* 'White Lady',
'White Queen'

Lavender: *Lavandula* × *intermedia* 'Edelweiss'

Lily of the valley: *Convallaria majalis*

Phlox: *Phlox drummondii* 'Isabellina'

Pink: *Dianthus* 'Chabaud Jeanne Dionis'

Snapdragon: *Antirrhinum majus* 'White Chantilly'

Sweet pea: *Lathyrus odoratus* 'Jilly'

White mignonette: *Reseda alba*

FILLERS

'Berggarten' sage: *Salvia officinalis* 'Berggarten'

Four o'clock: *Mirabilis longiflora* 'Fairy Trumpets'

Mint: *Mentha suaveolens* 'Variegata', 'Variegated Pineapple'

Scented geranium: *Pelargonium* 'Lady Plymouth', 'Nutmeg',
Pelargonium tomentosum 'Peppermint'

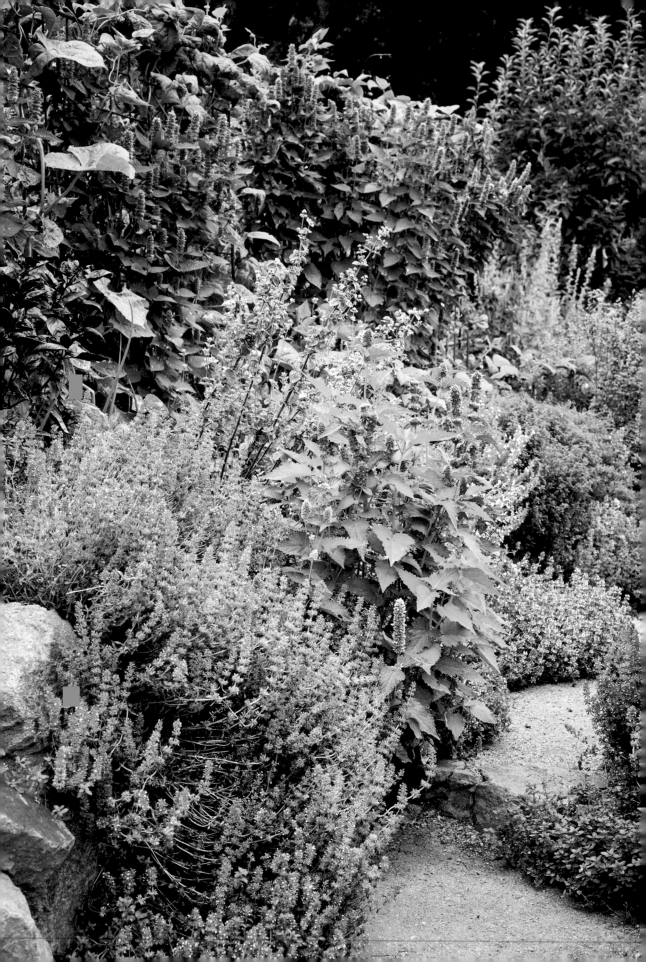

Culinary & Medicinal Gardens

Growing herbs is one of the most impactful things you can do in the garden. As some of the most fragrant plants in the garden, herbs can elevate your floral arrangements, salves, medicinal tinctures, cooking, and garden-grown teas. Fragrant herbs can be grown in containers, in dedicated planting beds, or in perennial beds. Planting herbs close together in the garden will help deter weeds and save water, and the area will be more attractive. Because you'll often harvest the herbs, you'll thin the bed as you harvest, so planting closer than the seed packet or plant tag suggests is okay.

In the front part of the dedicated bed, plant small and low-growing herbs such as thyme and cascading plants that will grow over the bed edging, such as 'Dwarf Greek' oregano and 'Wild Magic' basil. Fill out the center of the bed with medium-sized plants such as 'Honey Melon' sage (*Salvia elegans* 'Honey Melon') or feverfew (*Tanacetum parthenium*), and then place larger herbs in the back of the bed, such as lemon verbena (*Aloysia citrodora*) and scented geranium (*Pelargonium* 'Skeleton Rose'). Many herbs will produce flowers during their growing season. Let them bloom. The herb flowers add beauty to the garden, attract pollinators, and add to the garden's fragrance. Plus, they are edible. You can also tuck in fragrant perennials and annuals with edible flowers, such as hummingbird mint (*Agastache* spp.), calendula, chamomile, and alyssum.

Favorite edible fragrant flowers

In addition to chamomile, herb flowers, and roses:

Alyssum

Borage: *Borago* spp.

Calendula

Hummingbird mint: *Agastache* spp.

Lavender: *Lavandula* spp.

Lilacs: *Syringa* spp.

Nasturtiums: *Tropaeolum* spp.

Pinks: *Dianthus* spp.

Signet marigolds: *Tagetes tenuifolia* cultivars

Stock: *Matthiola incana*

Sweet violet: *Viola odorata*

anise hyssop, lemon thyme, French thyme, Greek oregano

Container Gardens

When space is limited, you can choose to grow plants in containers. Just be sure to choose plants that are well-suited for container plantings. Many annuals in cold-winter areas are perennials in gardens in warmer areas because they can survive the warmer winter temperatures. If you garden in an area with particularly cold winters, you can bring tender containerized plants indoors during the winter if you don't want to lose them to freezing temperatures. Great plants for containers include citrus, angel's trumpets (*Brugmansia* spp.), and frangipani (*Plumeria* spp.). If a container holds a large plant or shrub, go easy on your back and use a container dolly under the pot to wheel the container in and out.

The same principles of assessing your garden apply to container gardens. Know the soil, sun, and water conditions before selecting scented plants to include. Fill the container with a nutrient-rich organic potting soil and add granular organic fertilizer. Container plantings generally need more fertilization than in-ground plantings because nutrients are flushed through the container as you water and need to be replenished. Continue fertilizing the plants with either granular or water-soluble fertilizers monthly throughout the growing season. Choose plants that will be happy with the container's sun exposure. Containers can get hot very quickly on a sunny deck or patio, so make sure that shade-loving plants are in containers in shady locations. It's easy to set up a spigot-based irrigation system for plants in containers. If you plan to hand water your container garden, choose low-water plants that will be more forgiving if you miss a day.

Favorite fragrant plants for containers

Angel's trumpets: *Brugmansia* spp.

Citrus

Culinary and medicinal herbs (especially scented geraniums and mints)

Daffodils: *Narcissus* spp. or paperwhites: *Narcissus papyraceus*

Frangipani: *Plumeria* spp.

Freesias

Gardenias

Lavender: *Lavandula* spp.

Roses

Rosemary: *Rosmarinus officinalis*

stinking hellebore

BAD-SMELLING PLANTS (TO SOME)

Fragrance is subjective, but some flowers and plants are much admired for their botanical beauty, rather than their unpleasant odor. Whether it is a peony that smells like cat urine (not all varieties are pleasant smelling) or the stinking hellebore (*Helleborus foetidus*), these plants are lovable and fragrant, but not in a pleasant way.

Chameleon plant: *Houttuynia cordata*
Ginkgo (the female, seed producing tree)
Hellebores
Paperwhites: *Narcissus papyraceus*
Peonies: *Paeonia* spp.
Privets: *Ligustrum* spp.
Society garlic: *Tulbaghia* spp.
Spurges: *Euphorbia* spp.
Trilliums

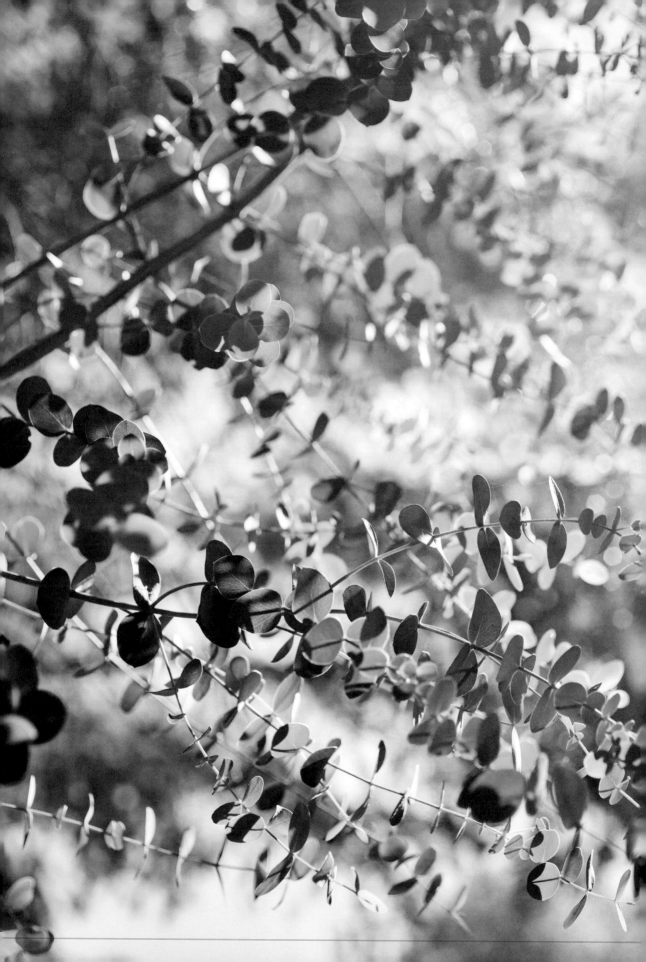

CHAPTER TWO

FAVORITE FRAGRANT PLANTS

This chapter explores fifty-five plants that can be included in a fragrant garden. This is not a comprehensive list by any means, but it includes plants for gardens in every USDA hardiness zone. Enjoy getting to know these fragrant plants, and take inspiration from them when you're planning your own garden space. Each profile includes the plant's scientific name, its common name, the hardiness zones in which it grows, its light requirements, ideal planting locales, and its scent profile.

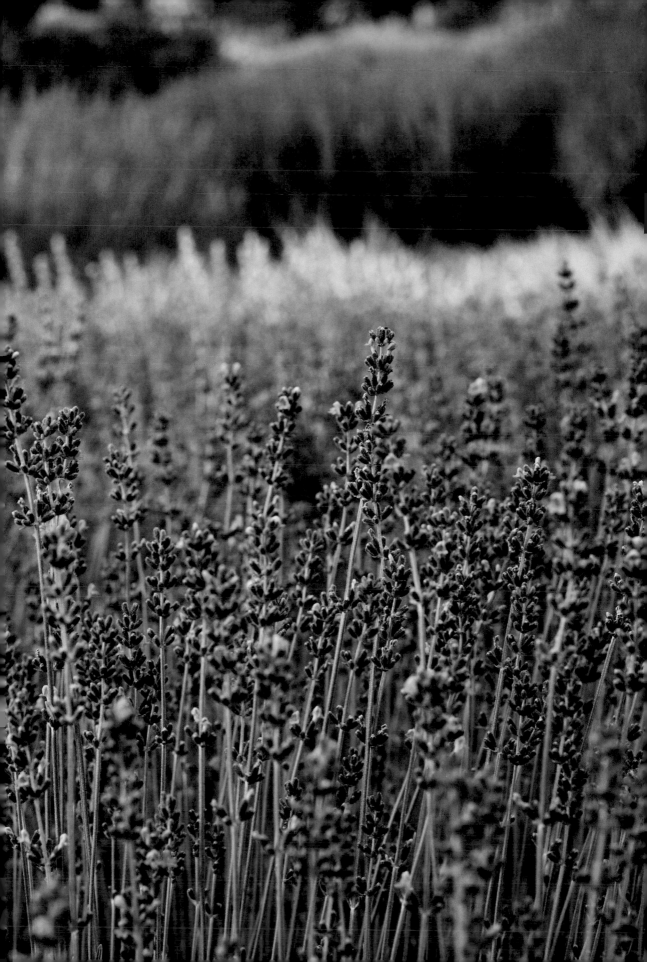

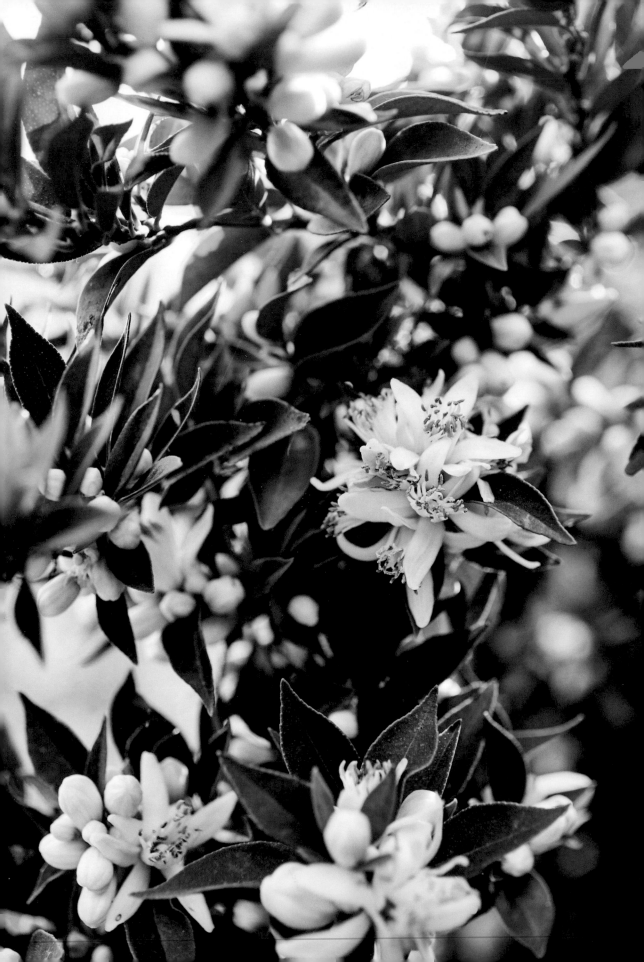

TREES

Citrus spp.

Citrus
Zones 9–11
Full sun

Landscapes, culinary and
medicinal gardens, containers
Tart, floral, spicy, acidic

In warm and tropical regions of the United States, citrus shrubs and trees have glossy, oval-shaped leaves year-round. The genus includes flowering and fruiting evergreen shrubs and trees with fragrant leaves, flowers, fruit, and fruit rind. A citrus tree or shrub creates one of the most recognizable and pleasing scents in the garden. Although the plant is often recognized by its powerfully scented flowers and fruit, even when it has neither it can still provide garden fragrance.

In spring, as you walk through your garden, you may smell citrus blossoms before you see them. Bees notice them too, as they happily zoom by on their way to visit the flowers. Citrus flowers are typically white with five petals. After the flowers have been pollinated, fragrant fruits begin to form.

Citrus is quite versatile in terms of growing requirements. Although the larger fruiting varieties need full sun, the smaller fruited, less sweet varieties such as lemons, limes, kumquats, and makrut limes will grow in partial shade, though they'll produce less fruit than when located in full sun. Be aware that many varieties have thorns along their branches. Place thorny trees in the middle of a planting bed or a large container, away from a high traffic area, to avoid passersby encountering the sharp thorns.

Frost protection is key with citrus. If area temperatures dip below freezing in the winter, keep citrus in containers so that you can move them inside for the winter, where they are protected. If frost is only an occasional issue where you live, frost blankets may be adequate to keep citrus safe during the winter.

All citrus varieties have amazingly scented leaves, flowers, and fruit, so you cannot go wrong. Choose a tree that is best suited for your garden. You can use citrus branches as a greenery base layer in fragrant arrangements. Branches with flowers or small fruits are great for large arrangements. Take branch

Chinotto orange

cuttings from mature trees. If you harvest from a younger tree, use smaller blossoms on small stems to add a gestural touch. Citrus with small fruits, such as kumquat (*Fortunella* spp.) and calamondin orange (*C.* × *mitis*), also make great additions to arrangements. Citrus flowers pair beautifully with amaryllis flowers in winter arrangements or with jasmine in spring arrangements.

Citrus—lemons in particular—can be used as a natural cleansing detoxifier: add lemon juice to vinegar to make a fragrant cleaning solution. Citrus is also a useful scent for the fragrance toolbox. The fruit's fragrant rind can be used to make perfume. It blends especially well with floral, woody, and spicy scents. Citrus flowers are also easy to use in perfumery. Note that when you harvest citrus flowers for arrangements and perfumery, you are forgoing the fruit harvest. So be sure to leave a few branches with flowers to develop into fruit.

Bergamot sour orange (*C. bergamia*): A beautiful blend of sweet and spice is the hallmark of the sour orange blooms.

Chinotto sour orange (*C.* × *aurantium var. myrtifolia*): Also known as myrtle-leaved orange, Chinotto is the basis for the fragrant Italian liquor Campari.

'Eureka' lemon (*C.* × *limon* 'Eureka'): with large spring flowers

Grapefruits: *C.* × *aurantium* 'Oroblanco', *C.* × *paradisi* 'Rio Red', with large, fragrant flowers

Makrut lime (*C. hystrix*): with fragrant foliage and flowers

Meyer lemon (*C.* × *meyeri*): with medium-sized flowers, citron/mandarin/pomelo hybrid

'Pink Lemonade' lemon (*C.* × *limon* 'Pink Lemonade'): with variegated green and white foliage, green and yellow striped fruit, pink flesh

'Chandler' pomelo (*C. maxima* 'Chandler'): with large, fragrant flowers

Eucalyptus spp.

Eucalyptus, gum tree

Zones 8–11

Full sun to part shade

Landscapes, gardens

Minty, camphor-honey, citrusy

Eucalyptus is a large genus that includes more than 500 species of shrubs and trees. It is part of the myrtle family. No matter the size of the plant, all eucalyptus have a similar camphor-honey fragrance, reminiscent of a cup of tea or a warm bath. Eucalyptus is a classic filler plant in arrangements and a must for the fragrant flower garden. Dwarf eucalyptus shrubs can be planted with lavender, ironwort (*Sideritis* spp.), and Cleveland sage (*Salvia clevelandii*) in the garden.

Wild eucalyptus trees can grow to more than 60 feet tall—far too large for a small garden space. There are, however, many shrubs and dwarf eucalyptus, though they will need pruning to keep them small—which is great, because this is a plant you will want to harvest often.

Include eucalyptus foliage in arrangements as filler at the edges of a vase to highlight the flowers. A single, long eucalyptus stem looks beautiful spilling from a vase, adding movement and fragrance to an arrangement. Versatile eucalyptus can be used for more than arrangements. Its boiled foliage is used to make a natural black dye that grows darker the longer it boils. Eucalyptus oil is traditionally used medicinally for respiratory ailments as an anti-inflammatory to enable better breathing. It also has a cooling effect for fever and sore muscles. Add a fresh stem to a hot bath, use it to make an oil infusion, or add it to an herbaceous flower tincture.

E. gunnii 'Silver Drop': annual for flower gardens, 2 to 3 feet tall

E. citriodora 'Lemon Bush': a favorite for citrus-scented arrangements

E. cinerea: silver dollar tree, with blue-green, coin-shaped leaves; good for container plantings and indoor arrangements

E. lunata 'Moon Lagoon': dwarf shrub for the dry, full sun landscape

Fruit trees

Zones 4–10

Full sun

Landscapes, culinary and medicinal gardens, orchards

Honey-like, floral

Fruit trees are at home in almost any garden, whether in a front garden or a backyard orchard. They also exude a lovely fragrance. Plant fruit trees in seasonal succession to have steady fragrance and fruit harvests throughout the year. Apricot, quince, apple, pear, peach, nectarine, and plum are favorite fragrant fruit tree choices for the home garden. The key to selecting the best tree for your garden is determining the area's growing conditions, especially regarding sunlight and access to water.

Fruit orchards are great additions to a backyard garden. You can underplant fruit trees with fragrant meadow flowers to attract pollinators to the trees' blossoms, creating a wonderfully scented space. Favorites for fragrant meadows include borage, yarrow, chamomile, hummingbird mint, lavenders, sage, scented geraniums, and perennial grasses. Create a pathway through the orchard to activate the subtle fragrance of the meadow plants as you brush against them. Add a sitting area where you can grab a book and relax.

When your fruit trees are in bloom, you can take a moment to stop and experience their scent. Apricots are some of the first to bloom, with honey-scented flowers. The scent of fruiting quince blossoms permeates the air with a highly fragrant, exotic fragrance that's similar to quince fruit.

If you're planting fruit trees in the front yard, place them away from sidewalks and driveways to avoid fruit falling on the cement. Fruit trees are usually pruned in late winter to promote growth and fruit development. You can also summer prune fruit trees to keep them at a manageable height for easy harvest. In the spring, prune and bring budding branches indoors and use them for gorgeous branch arrangements. The buds will bloom indoors!

peach tree

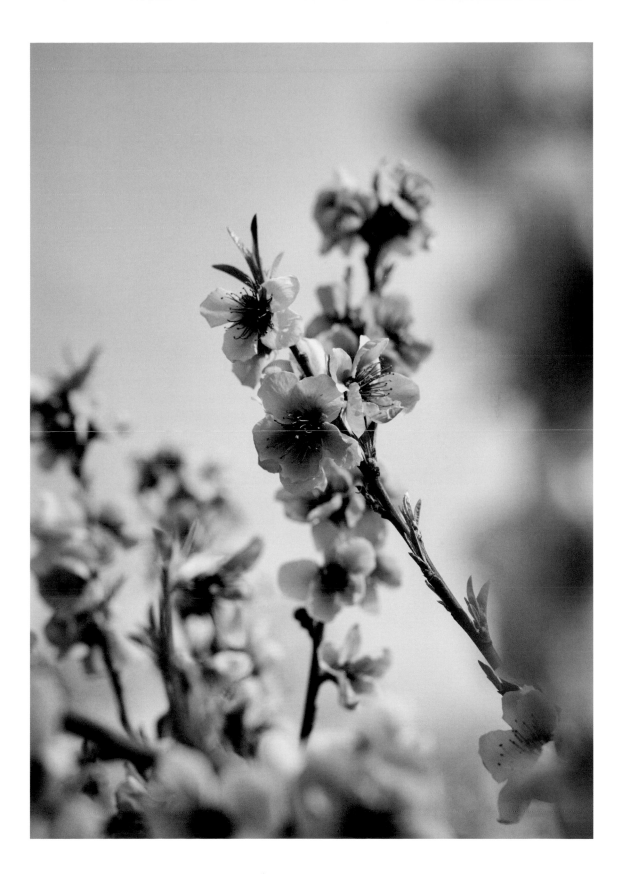

Laurus nobilis

Bay laurel, culinary sweet bay

Zones 8–11

Full sun to part shade

Landscapes, culinary and medicinal gardens, containers

Herbal, spicy, fresh, camphorous

A bay laurel will embellish your garden with its lush, evergreen foliage and refreshing, spicy-herbal fragrance. When planted in the ground, this sun-loving mediterranean garden staple requires little water after it's established. In areas outside its hardiness zones, bay laurel can be planted in a pot to move indoors during the colder months. A potted bay laurel requires regular, deep watering.

A bay laurel offers an aesthetically pleasing structure to a landscape and fits into almost any garden style. It can be used as a focal point, for screening, or as a hedge. This beautiful tree can grow to 60 feet tall at maturity, or it can be pruned into topiary shapes or maintained as a more natural shrub or tree in small gardens. Keeping it pruned to 8 feet or so makes it easier to harvest its fragrant branches.

Use fragrant bay laurel branches as a greenery base in arrangements, wreaths, and garlands. Its freshly cut, long, thin branches can be used to make wreath frames. Simply remove leaves and shape the branch into a circle, securing the ends of the branch with floral wire. The leaves' spicy scent blends well with many floral scents. It can also be added to flower tinctures along with rosemary and paperwhites or citrus blooms.

Magnolia champaca

Champak, joy perfume tree

Zones 9–10

Part shade

Landscapes

Sweet, spicy, floral

The heady fragrance of champak flowers, combined with roses and jasmine, is the basis for the expensive and exquisite perfume Joy, which is considered one of the greatest fragrances ever created. Formerly known as *Michelia champaca*, this handsome evergreen tree with large, lush, glossy green leaves grows in areas that receive no frost. Growing from 25 to 40 feet tall, this shade tree is adorned in yellow-orange, highly fragrant flowers from midwinter through spring, and they may often bloom sporadically through the summer as well. In the landscape, you may appreciate their fragrance before you see the tree.

Champak needs regular water and is not drought tolerant. It can be planted in full sun to shade; as the tree grows tall, its canopy will eventually be in full sun. Plant it at the back of the garden, where it has sufficient space to grow. If a champak is too large for your garden, consider a close relative, *Magnolia figo* (banana shrub), which is a tidier and more manageable plant than champak. This slow-growing evergreen shrub can be pruned and trained as a tree in hardiness zones 8 to 11. Its flowers are extremely fragrant, with a banana-like floral scent.

Champak's long blooming season makes it a fantastic addition to the fragrant garden. The star-shaped flowers are not very showy, but stems of foliage and blooms can be used as greenery base in arrangements. Use the flowers for enfleurage (extraction of essential oils) to create tinctures and oil-based infusions.

Olea europaea

Olive	Landscapes, containers
Zones 9–11	Clean, sweetly astringent, earthy and herbal
Full sun	

Fruiting olive trees probably aren't the first plants that come to mind when you are planning a fragrant garden. However, olive flowers have a beautiful herbal, clean scent that can be described as subtly warm, earthy, and sweetly astringent. We came across olive's fragrance by accident, as we were creating arrangements with flowering olive branches. Alethea smelled an amazing fragrance that was not coming from nearby flowers, but instead was from the blossoming olive.

The olive tree is a staple in the mediterranean garden. It provides screening and evergreen foliage, and it can be used as a stunning focal point. Olive trees can also be planted in large containers, although they must be watered more often than trees planted in the ground. There are fruiting and fruitless olive varieties, but if you are growing an olive tree for fragrance, you must plant the fruiting varieties, because the flowers create the fragrance. Site fruiting varieties away from concrete driveways and patios, where dropped fruit could cause staining.

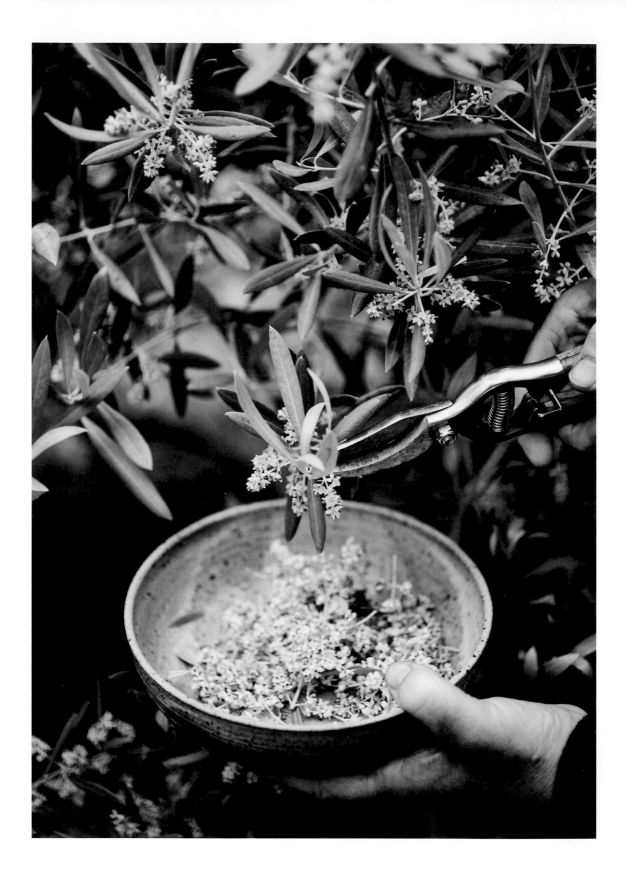

Olive branches can be used as foliage filler for arrangements or to form wreath bases, garlands, and swags. Olive flowers produce a clean, gender-neutral scent. Collect them to make essential oils, oil infusions, hydrosols (flower waters), and flower tinctures. Remember that when you harvest flowers, you are removing the parts that create fruit. Olives tend to fruit heavily every other year, so time your project with the tree's fruiting cycle so you can have your fruit and perfume too.

Plumeria spp.

Frangipani

Zones 10–12

Full sun

Landscapes, containers

Gardenia, honeysuckle, coconut

Frangipani flowers are showstoppers in the fragrant garden. In Hawaii, they are used in lei making. Their flowers instantly transport us to the islands—when you lean into a flower to breathe in its scent, you may want to hang out there for a while. It also grows in other areas with warm climates, including parts of California, Texas, and Florida. It is native to Latin, Central, and South America and the Caribbean and is fairly drought tolerant.

Frangipani can be grown as a shrub or small tree, as a focal point in the landscape, or in a large container. It has an open branch structure, and its star-shaped flowers appear on the tips of its branches in a wide range of colors. Although it won't tolerate freezing temperatures, don't give up on the idea of growing this fragrant powerhouse if you live in colder areas. If it's grown in a container, it can be overwintered indoors, and some folks even grow it in a sunny spot as a houseplant.

Flowers will bloom year-round in tropical climates, but where temperatures fall below 50°F, frangipani flowers will stop blooming and the plant will become winter deciduous (a trait we easily forgive once it starts blooming in spring). Red frangipani (*P. rubra*) fares better than most other *Plumeria* species in mainland gardens.

Harvest individual flowers for lei making or use small branches in arrangements. We use them for enfleurage natural scent extraction and for flower tinctures. The flowers' heady fragrance is easily captured in hydrosols and infusions as well.

olive flower harvest

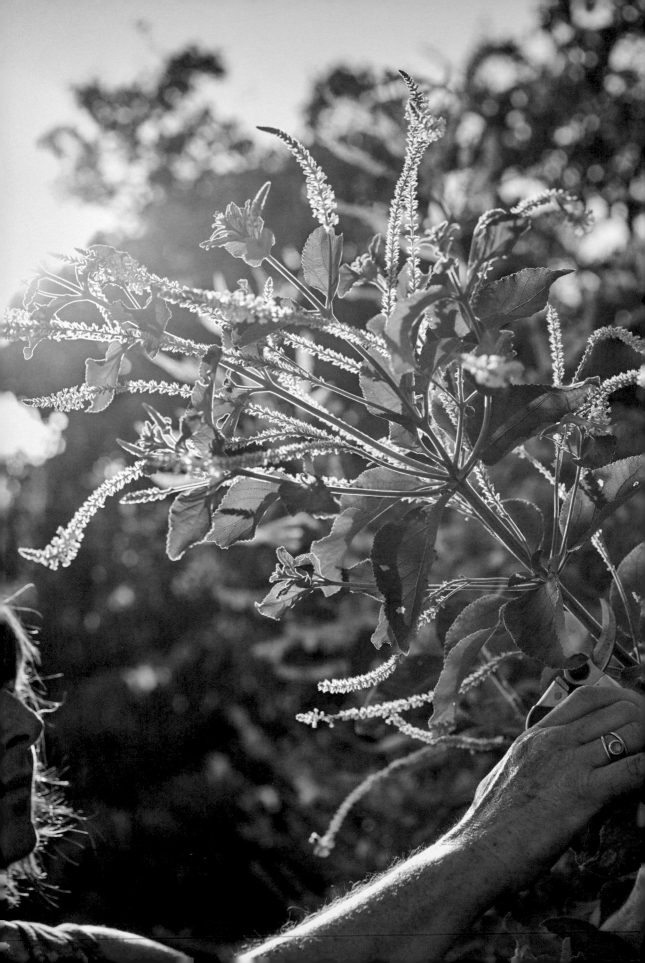

SHRUBS

Aloysia virgata

Sweet almond verbena, incense bush   Landscapes, containers
Zones 8–11   Almond, vanilla
Full sun

Sweet almond verbena has long, white spires of incredible vanilla- and almond-scented flowers that bloom from summer to fall. It is a must-have for fragrant gardens where it can be grown. You don't need to be up close to enjoy the flowers' aroma, which permeates the garden when these scent showstoppers are in bloom. Hummingbirds, butterflies, and bees love the flowers too.

This fast-growing, woody shrub or small tree prefers full sun but will tolerate part shade. In warm climates, it can be evergreen or semi-evergreen, whereas in colder climates, the plant is deciduous, dying back to the ground to await the next spring, when it may grow to 8 feet tall in one season! It's a great plant for fragrant hedgerows or fencerows, along with butterfly bush, lilacs, mock orange, and climbing roses. If you garden in colder climates, try growing sweet almond verbena in a container that you can bring indoors during winter months.

Make sure that you have easy access to the plants: because blooms form on new growth, pruning and harvesting blooming branches throughout the growing season will encourage more flowers in summer through fall. Unlike its cousin lemon verbena (*A. citrodora*), sweet almond verbena is not an edible plant. Instead, harvest it for arrangements and to use in natural scent projects. Its fast-growing nature makes it a great choice for including in large arrangements. Harvest branches when flowers first appear or are half open. Cut the branches in the morning and put them directly in water, keeping them out of direct sunlight to help prevent wilting. Use branches or flowers as a fragrant greenery base or secondary flower, mixing them with other herbaceous and floral-scented blooms. This verbena's unique almond fragrance brings out other floral notes in layered, mixed arrangements. Dry the flowers for scented projects including potpourri and wreaths. Sweet almond verbena also makes a great base scent for natural perfumes.

almond verbena

Brugmansia **spp.**

Angel's trumpets

Zones 7–11

Full sun

Landscapes, containers

Lily-like, tropical-floral, spicy, fruity, night-scented

In the evening, the trumpet-shaped flowers of this large plant have a spicy, tropical, intoxicating fragrance. Plant it outside your bedroom window to enjoy the aroma on a hot summer night, or use it near a hot tub or favorite nighttime gathering space. Sitting under the flowers in the late afternoon, just as they start to release their fragrance, and looking up into flowers backlit by the sun can be an intoxicating experience. This is a sexy plant.

The fragrant, pendent, trumpet flowers on this long-lived, soft, woody perennial can be from 4 to 24 inches long. This fast-grower can take the form of a shrub or a tree where it can be grown outdoors, blooming throughout the year. In cooler climates where it dies back in winter, it can grow up to 8 feet in a single season. A favorite cultivar, *B. × cubensis* 'Charles Grimaldi' has lush, handsome foliage and prolific apricot-colored blooms. *Brugmansia insignis* 'Betty Marshall' boasts beautiful white flowers and is considered the most winter-hardy cultivar (to about 25°F).

Angel's trumpets are sometimes confused with the short-lived perennial thorn-apples (*Datura* spp.), which also have fragrant, trumpet-shaped flowers. However, the flowers of thorn-apples are usually erect, while Angel's trumpets have pendent (suspended) flowers. Angel's trumpets are easy to grow from cuttings—a great way to share the plant with others. It's easily grown in a container as well as in the landscape and looks great with any lush or subtropical planting. Note that this plant is toxic if consumed, so as tempting as the scent may be, do not eat it!

Harvest a stem or branch in the late afternoon or evening when the plant is most fragrant and bring it indoors for a short-lived arrangement. The large flowers are also wonderful and dramatic for flower pressing. Enfleurage extraction is recommended for capturing their scent.

Buddleja spp.

Butterfly bush	Landscapes
Zones 5–9	Intensely sweet, fruity candy
Full sun	

The conical flower spires of butterfly bush bloom from spring through fall. Hardy and adaptable to many climates and soil types, this perennial shrub is a classic in cottage and flower gardens. Pollinators, including butterflies, are attracted to the flowers' nectar. Despite its name, however, butterfly bush is not a butterfly host plant—no butterfly larvae depend on the plant for nourishment. If you want to attract butterflies to stay and reproduce in your garden, include plants such as milkweed (especially for Monarch butterflies), fennel, and aster.

These shrubs are available in a wide array of selections and flower colors. *Buddleja davidii* 'Black Night' is a favorite for its dark purple blooms, and *B.* 'Hocus Pocus' has highly fragrant, cream-colored flower clusters. Seek out the harder to find *B. asiatica* (Asian butterfly bush), with white blooms that smell like freesias and that mix beautifully with other floral scents in a vase.

Butterfly bush is deciduous, but leaves emerge vigorously in the spring. Plant it toward the back of a bed or along a fence, where its bare branches won't detract from the garden during the winter months. It is also easily propagated from cuttings if you want to share plants with a friend. Note that butterfly bush can be invasive in certain parts of the world, where it grows vigorously. Make sure to check your areas' invasive plant species list before including it in your garden.

Harvest butterfly bush flowers in the morning when flower clusters are half open. The flowers are short lived in the vase, so cutting them from the garden makes more sense than buying them from a shop. Beautiful in single specimen arrangements or mixed with other blooms, butterfly bush flowers are heavily scented and can overpower other scents in a vase. Use it sparingly in natural scent projects when combining it with other scents—a few flowers go a long way.

Choisya ternata

Mexican orange,
Mexican orange blossom

Zones 7–10

Full sun to part shade

Landscapes, containers

Licorice, floral, orange blossoms

Mexican orange is one of our go-to fragrant-blooming shrubs when we need a background plant in the landscape. This evergreen winter and early spring bloomer is easy to grow, frost hardy, and tolerant of various soil types. It grows equally well in sun to partial shade. The white blossoms and foliage have a licorice-floral scent. It is native to the U.S. Southwest and Mexico, but it is not derived from citrus as its common name and scent implies.

This easygoing shrub is at home in any landscape style and makes a beautiful fragrant hedge or foundation planting. It boasts glossy, aromatic foliage, and its fragrant, white, star-shaped flowers are a winter and early spring nectar source for bees and butterflies. It also makes a great container plant and can be overwintered indoors in areas with colder winters. If its stems are pruned after flowering, the shrub may provide additional sporadic blooms during the summer.

Choisya × *dewitteana* 'Aztec Pearl' is a very profuse bloomer and is a bit more compact and less dense than *C. ternata*. *Choisya ternata* 'Sundance' is a great variety with chartreuse foliage that brightens a shady corner in the garden. The 'Sundance' cultivar, however, is not as forgiving as *C. ternata* and 'Aztec Pearl' when it comes to sun exposure, preferring morning sun or dappled light.

Mexican orange's pretty foliage and fragrant flowers add a beautiful base layer to arrangements. Its leaves and flowers add a subtle spicy scent and pair well with other floral fragrances in garden bouquets.

Mexican orange
blossom

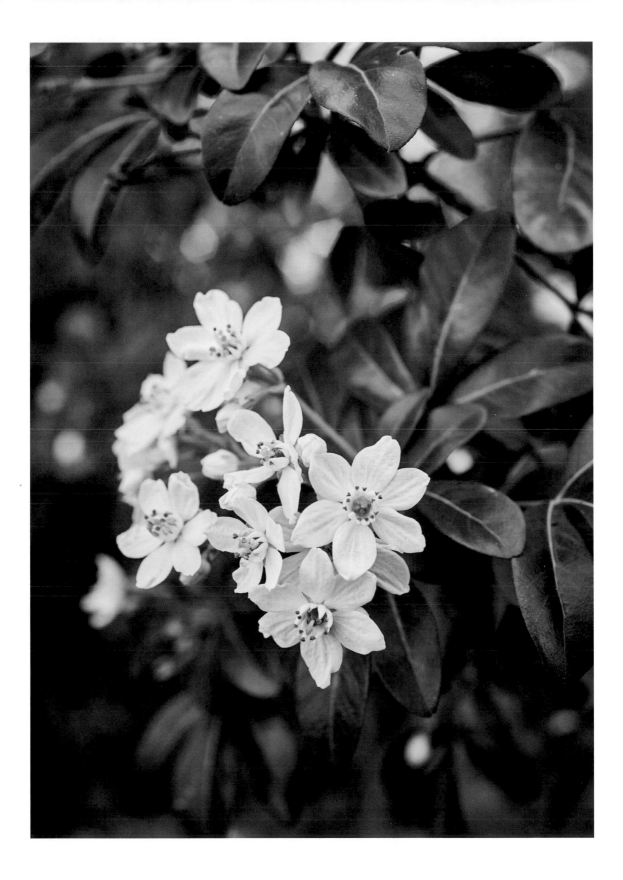

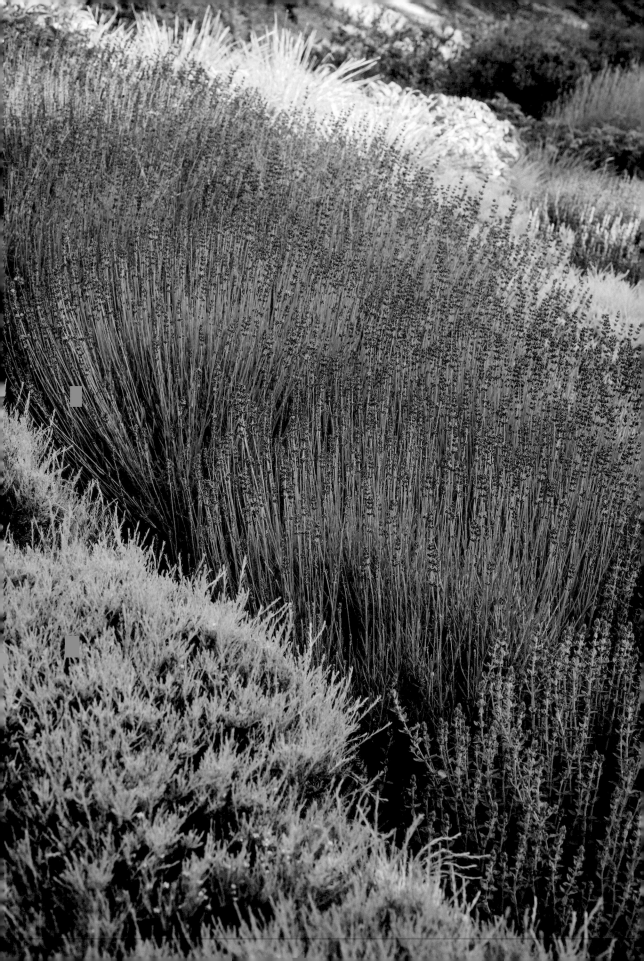

Coleonema pulchellum

Breath of heaven, confetti bush
Zones 8–12
Full sun to part shade

Landscapes
Tangy, citrusy

The common name of this fragrant evergreen shrub tells you all you need to know. Its brightly chartreuse, fragrant foliage contrasts nicely with silvers and purples in the landscape and looks fantastic with orange flowers if you want to turn up the heat a bit in your planting palette. Endearingly cheery, breath of heaven complements plantings of lavender, wall germander (*Teucrium chamaedrys*), and perennial grasses.

Every mediterranean garden needs a plant that is easy to grow, drought tolerant, and low maintenance, and breath of heaven offers it all. Although its pretty little pink flowers bloom throughout the growing season, this shrub is all about the foliage. Plant it along pathways, where you can brush up against it as you pass by and enjoy its luscious fragrance. Although not traditionally used in arrangements, its flowering stems make bright, feathery filler.

Daphne odora

Winter daphne
Zones 7–9
Full sun to part shade (prefers
morning sun and afternoon shade)

Landscapes
Floral, woody, vanilla

Daphne odora is one of the most unassuming shrubs in the garden, but it produces an amazing fragrance. One little sprig of winter daphne can fill an entire room with its sweet scent—it is the fragrance of a new year, and nothing smells quite like it.

In the garden, winter daphne can be a bit finicky when first planted. Depending on the time of year, we may lose up to 50 percent of our newly planted daphnes in the first year. The best time to plant it is in the fall through early spring. If it survives the first few months, it will be a low-maintenance and slow-growing evergreen shrub that prefers lower water once established.

breath of heaven,
'Hidcote' lavender

With unassuming green or silver foliage throughout most of the year, winter daphne is best tucked in a planting bed to support other plants, rather than being used as a focal point. It complements other dry-shade plants such as sweet box (*Sarcococca* spp.) and hellebores. In winter, its white, pink, or lavender flowers bloom in small clusters, often at the stem tips. Buds are dramatically pink before blooming, giving you a heads up that the fragrant blooms are about to arrive. Although summer-blooming daphnes are available, such as *D.* × *transatlantica* Eternal Fragrance, we always return to and plant winter daphne.

Harvest budding stems when half of the flower buds have opened. Daphne flowers are powerfully scented but unassuming and can easily get lost in a large arrangement. Nevertheless, single, small stems of flowers are worth adding to arrangements for their scent alone—or add a single sprig in a small vase on a bedside table or on a desk. Winter daphne is beautifully paired with winter foliage and other tiny blooms such as grape hyacinths (*Muscari* spp.) and violets. You can capture winter daphne's scent to enjoy all year long by creating flower tinctures and oil infusions using the enfleurage extraction method.

Gardenia jasminoides

Gardenia, cape jasmine

Zones 8–11

Full sun to part shade

Landscapes, cut flower gardens, containers

Spicy, zesty, tropical

The tropical scent of gardenia is a welcome addition to the landscape and cut flower garden. The exotic floral scent perfumes the entire garden in late spring and early summer. This broadleaf evergreen, flowering shrub is often planted in the landscape and in perennial beds surrounding dedicated annual cut flower beds.

Gardenias can be high maintenance, finicky plants. They need consistently moist, highly acidic, well-drained soil, and warm winters to bloom happily. In our hot and dry California summers, gardenias often struggle. Native to tropical Asia, gardenias prefer summer-moist climates, such as those found in the U.S. South, with regular rainfall. In gardens without summer rain, they can be planted in large containers, in acidic, well-drained soil with plenty of water. Planting in a container makes it easier to control water and soil conditions.

winter daphne

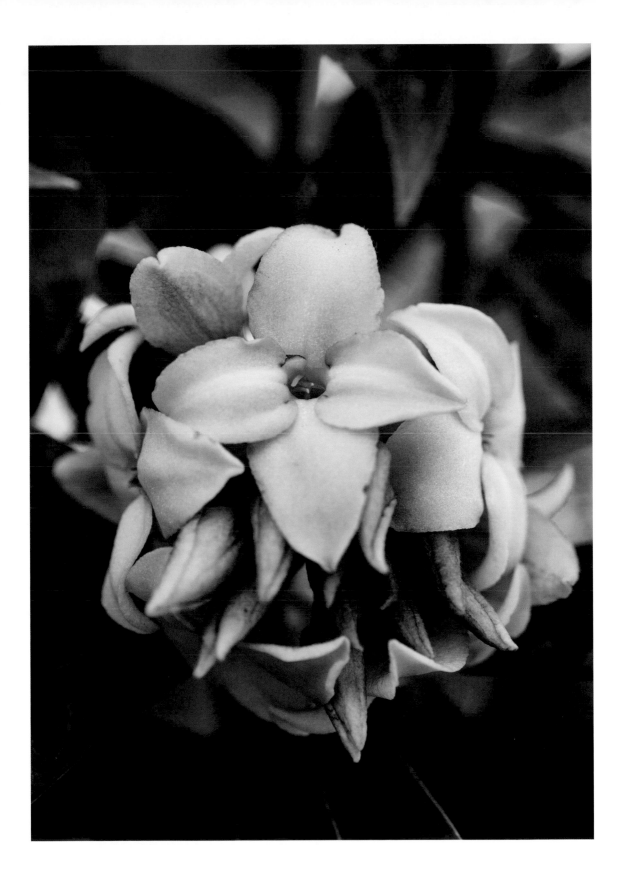

Single, semidouble, or double white flowers bloom from late spring to early summer, with a beautiful, heady, tropical fragrance. Its glossy, dark green foliage is attractive in the garden even when the gardenia is not in bloom. It can be part of a foundation planting, a low hedge, or a border planting.

When using gardenias in arrangements, because their flowers face downward, they need to be propped up by other flowers or foliage. This classic corsage flower is easy to use in preserving projects because it delivers a lot of scent. Gardenia's warm and sexy, timeless fragrance is commonly used in perfumes.

Lavandula spp.

Lavender	Landscapes, culinary and medicinal gardens, containers
Zones 5–9	
Full sun	Floral, herbal, sweet, woodsy

With one of the most recognized fragrances in the world, lavender generously offers many culinary, medicinal, and decorative uses. The flowers can be the fragrant foundation of garden wreaths, oil infusions, and flower tinctures. In the kitchen, lavender can be used to flavor salt and sugar—and it makes a good cup of tea.

Lavenders vary in size and flower color and can be used in almost any application in the landscape. They are drought-tolerant, evergreen, pollinator attracting perennials with fragrant foliage and flowers. In areas outside its preferred hardiness zones, it is well worth growing as an annual.

Some favorites for the fragrant garden include larger varieties such as *L.* 'Goodwin Creek Gray' and *L.* × *intermedia* 'Provence', 'Grosso', and Phenomenal. Good smaller varieties include *L. angustifolia* 'Hidcote', and 'Munstead', and the white-flowering *L.* × *intermedia* 'Edelweiss'. Lavender lasts a good ten years in the garden and then needs to be replaced. Look for plants in 4-inch or 1-gallon pots in the nursery, and stay away from larger specimens that will expire more quickly.

Harvest lavender stems in the cool morning when they are fresh and when flowers are just beginning to open. Use a few stems bunched together in arrangements rather than placing them singly so that the flowers create more visual impact. Lavender can be a gestural touch when used as secondary

lavender harvest

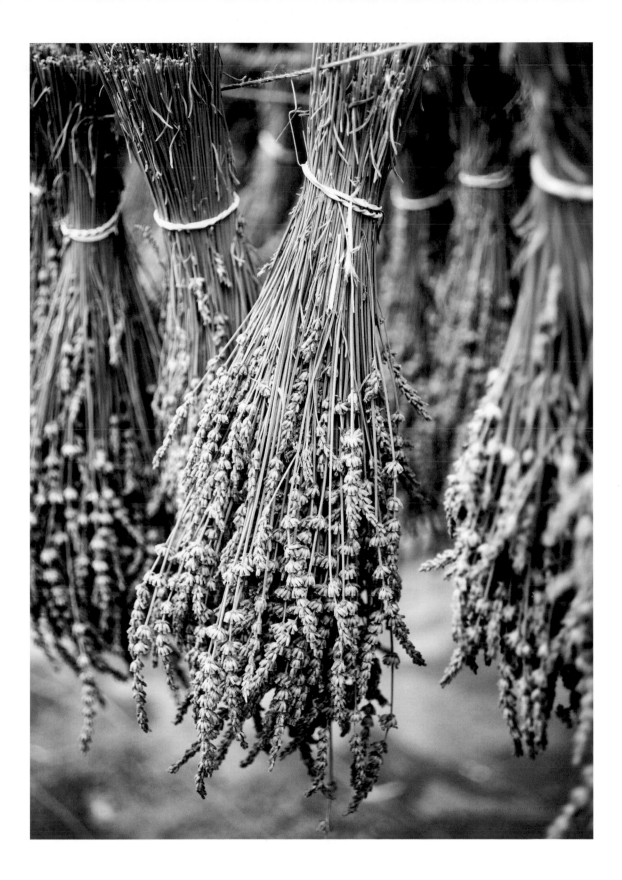

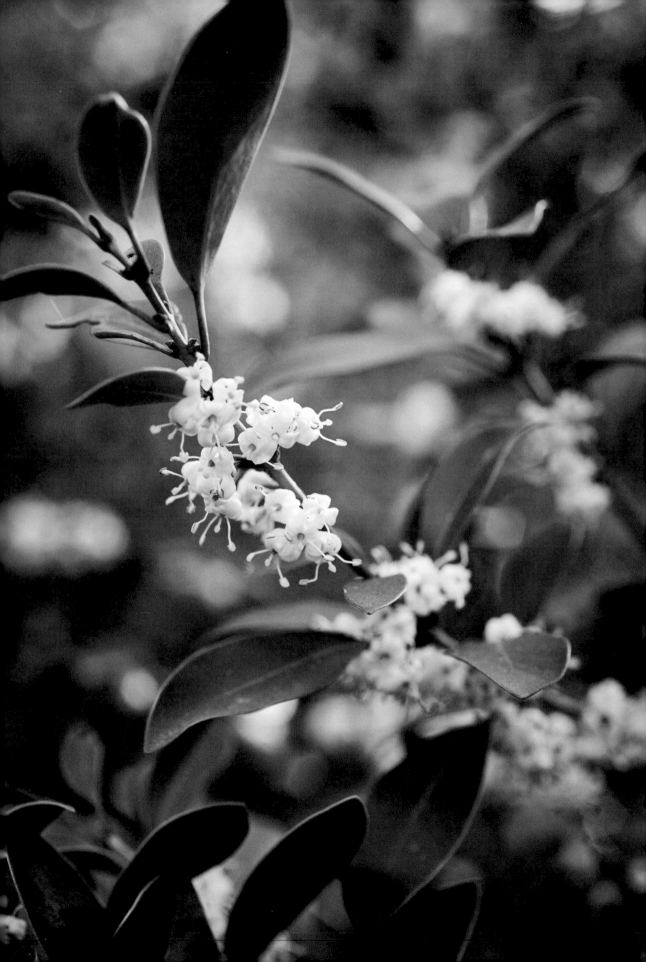

flowers in an arrangement, or it can be used to fill an entire vase. You can also use bunches of lavender stems and flowers to make a large, Tuscan-inspired arrangement. If you have a large harvest, make a lavender wreath.

When harvesting lavender for natural scent projects, include both foliage and flowers because the plant's essential oils are derived from both. As you use your creations through the winter, they will remind you of warmer days to come. Lavender's scent pairs well with roses and citrus but can overpower other fragrances, so it needs a bold partner in arrangements and perfumery. Be careful using it in skin products because some people suffer from allergic reactions to the essential plant oils. In many projects, a little goes a long way. Use lavender hydrosol as a pillow spray for kids to calm anxieties before sleeping—it provides a scented clue that bedtime is soon. Lavender potpourri can fill a small room with fragrance or can be added to a soothing bath. Calming and reflective, the scent of lavender invokes memories of warm summer days.

Osmanthus fragrans, O. heterophylus

Sweet osmanthus, holly olive	Landscapes
Zones 7–9	Vanilla, floral, freesia
Full sun to part shade	

If you need green foliage to hide an ugly fence or screen out your neighbor's property, osmanthus is the answer. This great backdrop plant is also a wonderfully fragrant blooming shrub and can be used to create a fragrant garden wall. Petite white blooms fill the garden with a soft but heady fragrance. The evergreen shrub is a relatively maintenance-free favorite for a side yard screen planting or at the back of the garden along a pathway. Because osmanthus is a slow grower, you can wait to prune it until you harvest stems and larger branches to use in an arrangement. *Osmanthus fragrans* blooms twice a year in the spring and fall, and *O. heterophylus* blooms in the late fall to early winter.

Use its flowering, leafy branches in arrangements, where its stems have a pretty shape and add movement. Tuck winter-blooming osmanthus stems in wreaths; the flowers will remain scented even when dried. Or simply dry and preserve the flowers to add to garden sachets, potpourri mixes, and tinctures.

sweet osmanthus

Paeonia spp.

Peony	Landscapes, cut flower gardens
Zones 3–8	Fresh and floral, or cat urine and
Full sun	stale fish (selection dependent)

Billowy, multipetaled, and romantic peonies are some of the most beloved spring flowers in the garden—at least until you put your nose in them. A peony can send up a fresh, floral scent that perfumers worldwide synthesize to make perfumes. On the other hand, if you are unlucky enough to sniff a cultivar like *P.* 'Coral Charm' (a florist favorite), you may quickly be repelled by the off-putting aroma of cat urine or stale fish.

In the garden, some plants have a built-in defense system that keeps them safe from predators. Our favorite roses, for example, are often the thorniest ones, capable of repelling deer and rabbits from eating them (sometimes). We hypothesize that peonies, likewise, have evolved to defend themselves from florists and gardeners, who would otherwise hoard all of the plants' blooms! Why else would a plant so beautiful smell so bad? In all seriousness, do your homework before choosing a peony for the fragrant garden. There are many cultivars to choose from, but only some are pleasantly fragrant, including these: *P. lactiflora* 'Chestine Gowdy', 'Cora Stubbs', 'Duchesse de Nemours', 'Hermione', and 'Sarah Bernhardt'. Fragrant Itoh peonies, which are crosses between herbaceous and tree peonies, include cultivars 'Bartzella', 'Cora Louise', and 'Julia Rose'.

A great way to identify the best peonies for your garden is to visit a local botanical garden or plant nursery. Stroll through the gardens or aisles and take time to smell the individual peonies that speak to you visually, ensuring they will be a pleasant addition to your fragrant garden.

Harvest peonies in the morning, just as the blooms are about to open and each bud looks similar to a large, fluffy marshmallow. Blooming peonies last a good week in a vase. These large focal flowers need to be given space in the vase, especially because the flowers will continue to open over the lifetime of the arrangement. Keep this in mind as you choose secondary flowers to complement peonies in your arrangements, as smaller blossoms can get lost behind them. We capture and preserve peonies' scent with all of the infusion techniques, especially enfleurage.

'Julia Rose' peony

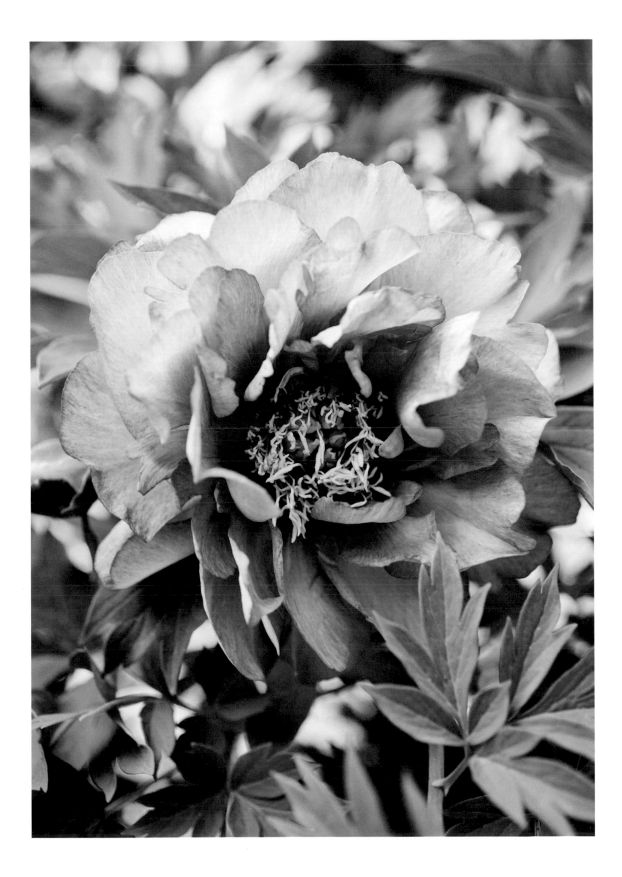

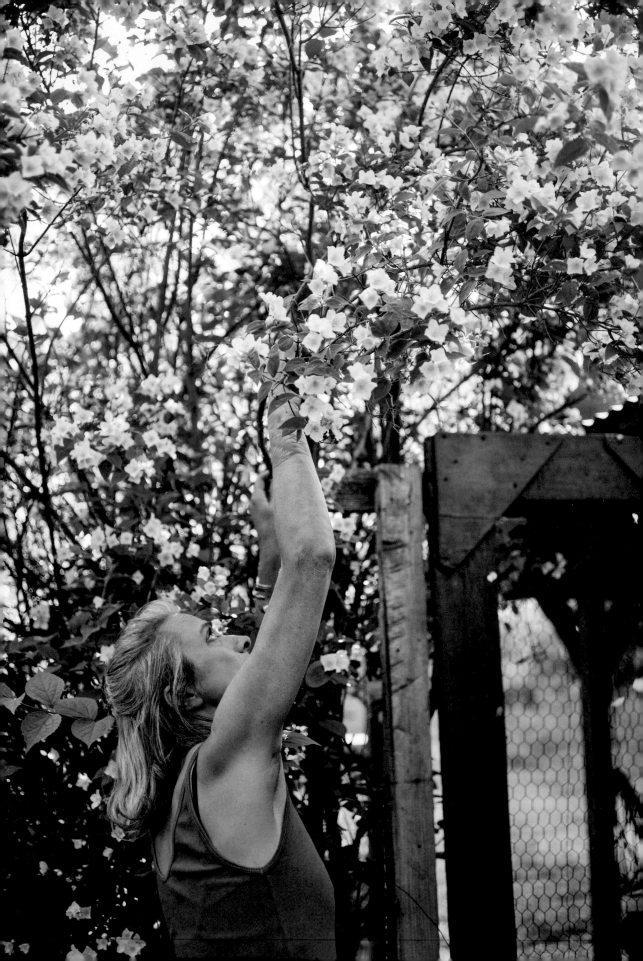

Philadelphus spp.

Mock orange

Zones 4–8

Full sun to part shade

Landscapes, cut flower gardens

Floral, citrus, ambrosia

Monstrous and wild in all of the best ways, mock orange is a flowering shrub that makes a big fragrance impact. From late spring to early summer, long before you see its beautiful white flowers, you'll know it is in bloom by the fragrance in the air.

This shrub wants to grow large, so give it lots of room. Combine mock orange shrubs with lilacs and climbing roses at the back of a garden bed to create a fragrant hedgerow. By placing these deciduous shrubs in the back of the bed instead of front and center in the garden, their winter-bare branches won't be as noticeable. When not winter-dormant, mock orange makes a good screening hedge, and it is beloved by butterflies and bees. Most plants need regular water, while Lewis' mock orange (*P. lewisii*) is drought tolerant once established.

Harvest large branches from mature shrubs for stunning and dramatic late spring/early summer arrangements. Choose stems with half of their flowers open and the other half budded up. Because this is a woody shrub, you'll need to make a diagonal cut on the stem to enable the branch to absorb more water in the vase. Directly after cutting branches, if possible, put them in a bucket of water overnight before using them in an arrangement. You can use big, ambrosia-scented branches on their own as a single statement piece or harvest smaller stems to mix with other late-spring garden flowers such as lilacs and roses. Once the shrub is done blooming, the foliage is so pretty that its stems can be used as greenery. Mock orange's fragrance is wonderful on its own or when included in floral/citrus blends for natural perfume. Because the flowers grow so large, you will have plenty on hand for making hydrosols, tinctures, and enfleurage.

mock orange

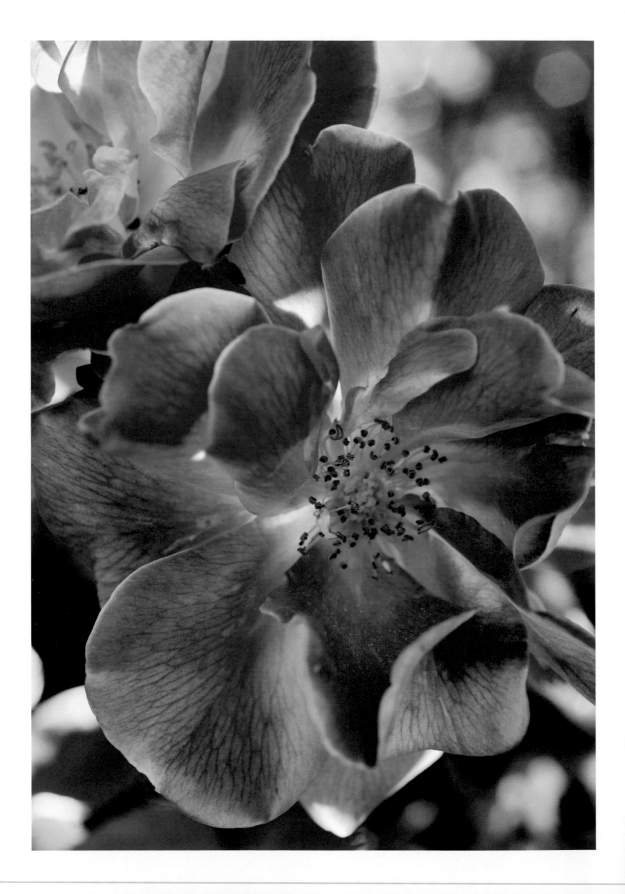

Rosa spp.

Rose

Zones 3–10 (selection dependent)

Full sun to part shade (selection dependent)

Landscapes, cut flower gardens, culinary and medicinal gardens, containers

Fruity, myrrh, spicy, tea, musky

Roses are plants with emotive qualities. Many of us reminisce about the roses in our grandparents' garden or a first bouquet from a special friend. With a wide variety of colors, scents, and tastes, roses offer what few other plants can. A rose releases its fragrance when it is mature and ready for pollination—typically when flowers are half open and in the morning. Although roses have a familiar fragrance, not all roses are fragrant. Many have been bred for durability and appearance, losing their scent in the process. Generally, English roses and old roses are the most fragrant. Read the plant label at the nursery, check online, or talk to knowledgeable gardeners or nursery staff before purchasing a rose for your fragrant garden.

Roses can fill many spaces in the garden. They can be used as ground covers, shrubs, climbers, or container plants. Though most roses prefer full sun, some cultivars can grow in part shade. Most of these hardy perennials can survive in a variety of growing conditions. (In fact, the world's oldest living rose, the Rose of Hildesheim in Germany, is believed to be a thousand years old!) With many different types and cultivars to choose from, keep hardiness in mind when acquiring roses for your garden. Some varieties are finicky, while others are so low maintenance that you can simply plant them along a fence and let them ramble. Some roses are happy in containers. Placement is also important when it comes to adding roses to the garden, especially because of thorns, though thorniness can vary greatly. Avoid placing a particularly thorny variety along a slender pathway, where passersby may be "bitten."

Roses have specific blooming cycles. Some have only a single bloom period, while others will bloom throughout the growing season. If you plant several types of roses with different bloom times, your garden can be filled with colorful blooms from spring through fall. The more you deadhead your roses when flowers are done blooming, the more they will send up new growth to begin again. Every month during the growing season, feed roses with fish emulsion to encourage new growth.

'Joseph's Coat' rose

The rose is the queen of the flower world. In arrangements, roses can serve as focal or secondary flowers, depending on the flower shape and size. They are also the basis of many fragrant products. Rosewater, rose toner, rose salve, rose tincture—you can use roses for a variety of homemade products, though it can take up to 60,000 petals to extract a single ounce of essential oil. For the home fragrance gardener, it is all about the hydrosol and oil infusions. If you have a favorite rose scent profile, include multiple varieties of roses with similar scents to ensure that you have plenty of plant material to work with.

Many of the most fragrant roses are also the thorniest. Perhaps this is nature's way of keeping deer and humans alike from greedily harvesting all of the plant's blooms before the bees have a chance to pollinate them. Choosing a single favorite rose variety is nearly impossible, but our favorites tend to be Old English roses such as these.

'Cecile Brunner': climbing rose with profuse, sweet-smelling, pale pink blooms

Emily Brontë ('Ausearnshaw'): soft cream-apricot flowers, large repeating blooms, strong tea/old rose scent

Eustacia Vye ('Ausegdon'): pink blooms, strong fruity scent

The Generous Gardener ('Ausdrawn'): pale pink climbing rose, repeating blooms, old/myrrh/musky scent

Munstead Wood 'Ausbernard': deep crimson-red blooms, strong old rose/fruity scent

Rosmarinus officinalis

Rosemary
Zones 7–10
Full sun

Landscapes, culinary and medicinal gardens, containers
Strong, camphorous, woody, balsamic

Aromatic and evergreen, with blue flowers and a soothing fragrance, rosemary is useful and beautiful, and perfect for hedges and structure in the garden. From late winter through spring and summer, blue or white flowers brighten the garden.

Rosemary can be grown in herb gardens, in borders, or as foundation plantings, but it can take on a variety of roles in the garden, from an ornamental

'Tuscan Blue' rosemary

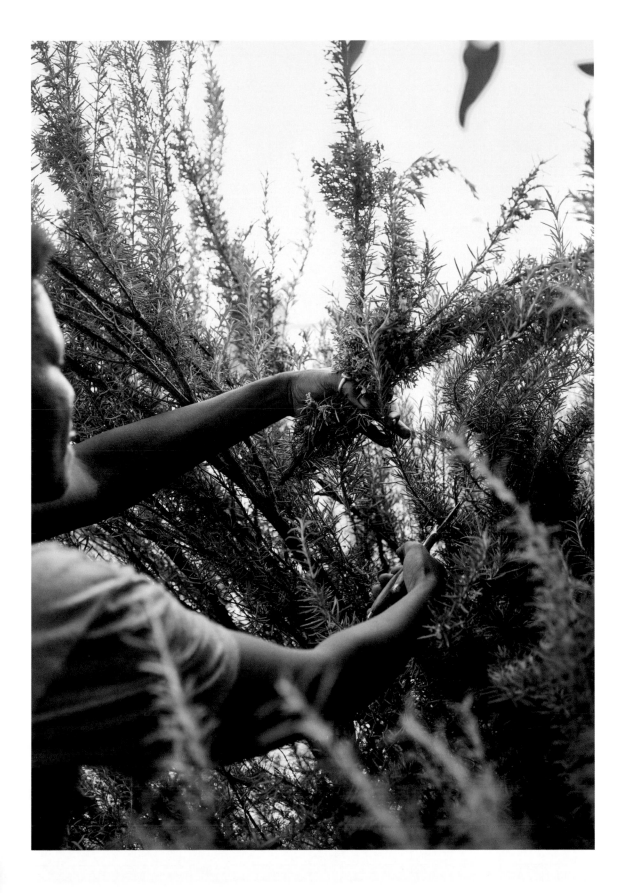

specimen plant to a low hedge. Container plantings bring its beautiful scent to patios, decks, and any other sunny areas. In colder areas where needed, you can grow rosemary in a container and overwinter it indoors.

Rosemary can serve as greenery in winter arrangements, and it can be used as a wonderful base for a scented wreath, with or without its needle-like leaves. Branches can be easily bent and turned to make a wreath base with simple floral wire. Whether used in a vase or in a perfume, rosemary pairs well with paperwhites and citrus scents. We also love the scent of rosemary on pets—especially our otherwise stinky dogs. Place it in gardens where your dogs can visit and rub against it. We also like to make rosemary vinegar infusions as an all-purpose cleaner for countertops and surfaces that aren't dogs.

Salvia clevelandii

Cleveland sage, fragrant sage	Landscapes
Zones 8–11	Sage, musky, earthy, pungent
Full sun	

Salvia clevelandii is the fragrance of California heat and the state's dry wildland, the chaparral. If you garden in a mediterranean climate, this is the sage for you. This California native is an extremely drought-tolerant plant and a gardening go-to for those who live where water needs to be conserved. It's also a go-to plant for pollinators such as hummingbirds, butterflies, and bees.

Like all sages, Cleveland sage is in the mint family. Its fragrant foliage isn't minty, but is more similar to its cousin, culinary sage. It has beautiful blue-violet flowers in spring and early summer and gray-green foliage. When it's done blooming, resist the urge to prune, because the dried flower spikes provide beautiful visual interest in the garden throughout fall—the best time to prune this plant.

This subshrub grows 2 to 5 feet tall and wide in many types of well-draining soil. For a beautifully dramatic landscape, plant Cleveland sage en masse on a hillside or mixed with grasses, white sage (*S. apiana*), and yarrow (*Achillea* spp.) in a meadow. Smaller cultivars such as 'Winifred Gilman' are suitable for smaller beds and gardens, as long as they are planted in full sun and with other waterwise plants.

Dried bracts keep their scent and are fantastic in dried arrangements and wreaths. Add leaves to hydrosols when making a cleansing medicinal scent.

Sarcococca spp.

Sweet box	Landscapes
Zones 6–9	Sweet vanilla
Part shade to shade	

Few plants have a more appropriate common name than sweet box. This evergreen shrub has glossy, green leaves and fragrant, wispy, white flowers, with berries appearing in late winter and early spring. It is a problem-solver for the most difficult garden space—dry shade—and its roots tolerate a range of soils. The flowers of this late winter to spring–blooming shrub have an unusual, heady vanilla fragrance that fills the garden, and birds love the berries. Combine it with fellow fragrant and dry-shade growers, hellebores and winter daphne, in a beautiful woodland planting. The most commonly available selections include a shrub form, fragrant sweet box (*S. ruscifolia*), and low-growing Himalayan sweet box (*S. hookeriana*).

A little goes a long way when using sweet box in a vase. Snip a stem or two for a small, intimate arrangement to place near your bedside or favorite reading spot. Add its blooms to flower tinctures and combine them with other floral scents in oil-based infusions.

Syringa vulgaris

Lilac	Landscapes, cut flower gardens
Zones 3–7	Intensely sweet, spicy
Full sun	

Few scents are more synonymous with spring than lilac flowers, which bloom for an intense but brief period. Think of these fragrant flowers as your spring fling. For a couple of weeks, lilac will be the star in the fragrant garden. Then, for the rest of the year, it is a nondescript, woody, deciduous shrub.

Lilacs' singularly strong, stand-alone scent is emotive, and it reminds many of us of our grandmothers' gardens. They bloom in shades of purple, pink, and white. Bicolor varieties (white and purple or white and pink) are also available. Although the flowers are fleeting, it is possible to prolong the fragrant flowering

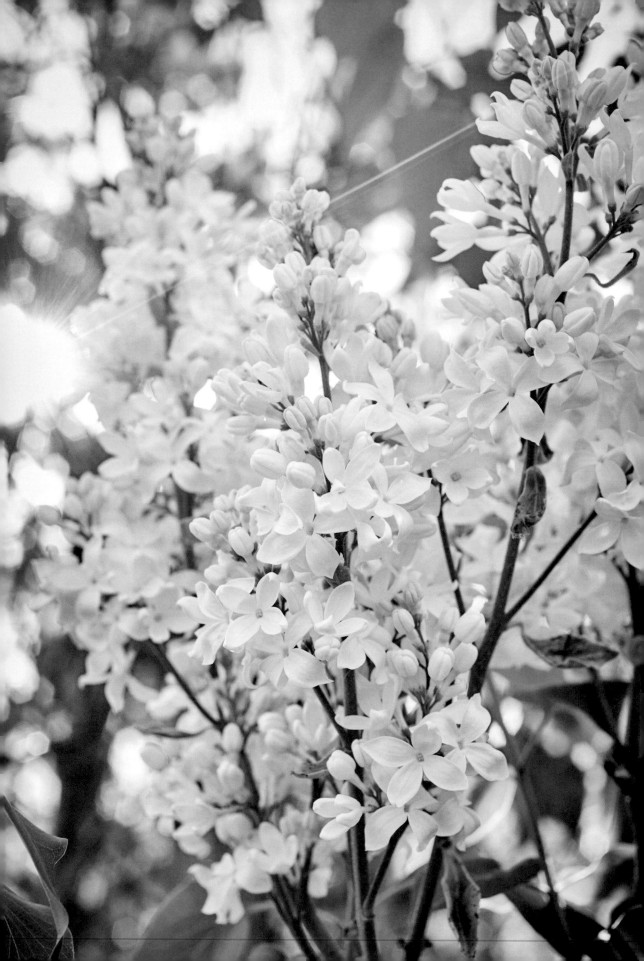

season by planting selections with early, middle, and late bloom times. Because their blossoms are short lived, lilacs aren't best used as focal points for a cut flower garden or a landscape. Place them toward the back of a garden, along a fence, or in other spots in full sun.

Lilac flowers can be heavily harvested. In the vase or garden, these flowers are the stars, as their colorful flowers fill out an arrangement and their fragrance fills the air. Lilac foliage makes great greenery bases in arrangements.

For natural scent projects, lilacs combine well with most spring flower fragrances. Use them in a spring flower blend or alone as an enfleurage, flower tincture, or oil infusion. You can do anything with lilac flowers—but quickly.

Viburnum carlesii

Korean spice viburnum	Landscapes, cut flower gardens
Zones 4–7	Sweet, spicy, vanilla
Full sun to part shade	

Viburnum carlesii is one of the great early spring–bloomers in the fragrant cottage garden. Slow growing but reliable, its heady, vanilla-scented flowers grow in clusters resembling snowballs that appear just as the snow is melting.

Korean spice viburnum is an easygoing shrub, which makes it a great choice for a fragrant foundation or hedge planting. Because it likes regular, even watering, it is not a good choice for low-water gardens. Though it can reach 6 feet tall, its slow-growing nature makes it low maintenance. If you need to prune a viburnum, the best time is immediately after it blooms, because the following year's buds develop in the summer, and you can risk cutting off next year's flower harvest if you prune later. If two varieties are in the garden, their flowers can cross-pollinate, resulting in berries that are much loved by birds.

Harvest branches for arrangements or other uses just as the flower heads are beginning to open in early spring. As with other woody plants, cutting stems at an angle enables them to absorb more water in the vase. Harvested viburnum branches also benefit from conditioning—placing them in a water-filled bucket in a cool, dark room for at least five hours before they are used in arrangements. The pink to red buds open to white flower clusters that complement other spring bloomers in a vase. The scented blooms are

'Angel White' lilac   wonderful in floral and citrus blends for infusions and tinctures.

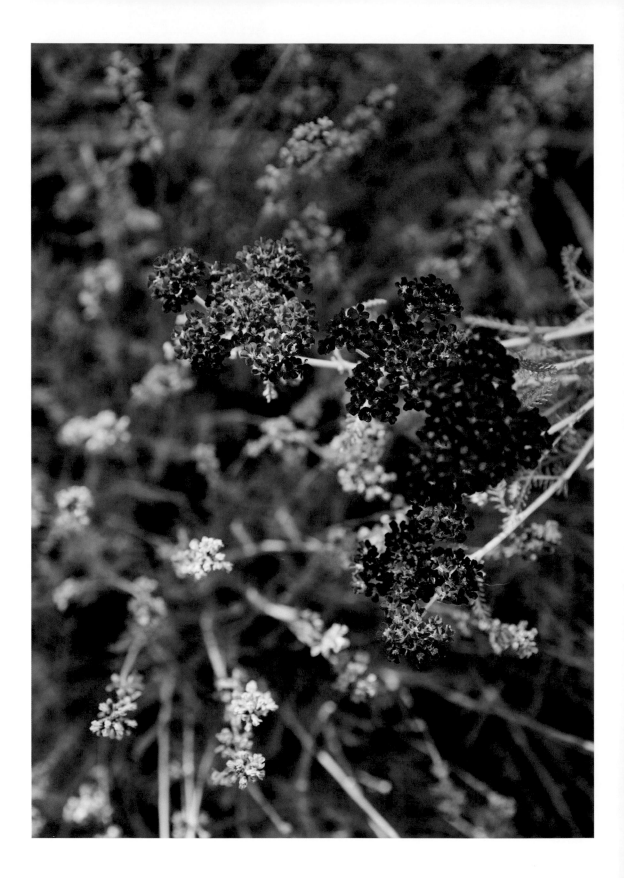

PERENNIALS

Achillea millefolium

Yarrow

Zones 3–9

Full sun

Landscapes, cut flower gardens, culinary and medicinal gardens, containers

Pungent, musky, herbal

Although often planted as a flowering perennial, yarrow can be a valuable herb in the garden because of its durability as well as its medicinal uses. Hardy and versatile, with fernlike leaves, yarrow's large, colorful, flat-topped flower clusters are beautiful in any garden. Yarrow's scent is not for everyone, however. This medicinal plant's fragrance is strong, sharp, and pungent.

Yarrow attracts many beneficial insects to the garden, including butterflies, moths, and bees. Hardy in any soil type, it thrives in full sun with low water. Snip spent blooms throughout the summer to stimulate continuous blooming. In fall, once it is done flowering, cut the spent flower stems to the ground. Yarrow is available in a wide array of colors. In a cut flower garden with a dusky palette, try 'Apricot Delight', 'Terracotta', and other muted peach-colored and pastel cultivars. 'Pomegranate' is a favorite deep red cultivar, and A. 'Moonshine' has gray foliage and bright yellow blooms.

Yarrow's fernlike foliage lends a beautiful texture to arrangements, and its broad flower heads can be used as a secondary or filler ingredient. Yarrow also pairs beautifully with coneflowers (*Echinacea* spp.), bee balms (*Monarda* spp.), and sage (*Salvia* spp.) in a wildflower-inspired arrangement. Use dried and preserved stems of yarrow flowers in darker and more saturated colors for arrangements and wreaths, as pale yarrow flower colors do not hold up well when dried. Yarrow's antibacterial, anti-inflammatory, astringent, and analgesic qualities make it a wonderful scented addition to fragrant medicinal hand salves and tub mixes. Pair it with strong floral scents.

'Pomegranate' yarrow, 'Hidcote' lavender

Agastache spp.

Hummingbird mint

Zones 4–10

Full sun

Landscapes, culinary and medicinal gardens

Licorice, minty, floral

With flowers in almost every color and plants ranging from 18 to 36 inches tall, every garden should include hummingbird mint. Its variety makes it one of the most versatile of the fragrant plants in the landscape. This scented plant gives and gives at every stage of its life—from its aromatic leaves to its edible flowers and seeds.

Anise hyssop (*A. foeniculum*) is a culinary plant in the genus. Plant it along trellises and in planting beds in the kitchen garden to attract pollinators to annual vegetables; in herb gardens to add beautiful, tall spikes of light purple blooms; and in perennial beds, mixed with other fragrant, edible, and cut flowers such as feverfew (*Tanacetum parthenium*), coneflowers, and bee balms. Cultivars 'Blue Boa' and 'Tutti-frutti', and *A. aurantiaca* 'Apricot Sprite' are just a few favorites to plant throughout the garden.

A must for a dry garden, hummingbird mint will also thrive if it receives plenty of water. Its nectar-filled flowers are constantly visited by hummingbirds, finches, and bees and are sturdy enough to support a perching bird. It blooms throughout summer and fall, and if flowers are harvested in early summer, a second flush of blossoms can continue until the first frost. After frost, the deciduous plants will die to the ground, reemerging in spring.

Harvest anise hyssop leaves from early spring through fall. Its prolific floral spikes add a great wispy touch to summer arrangements, and it dries well for wreaths. Its minty and floral scents add an herbaceous touch to garden arrangements and perfumery projects.

anise hyssop

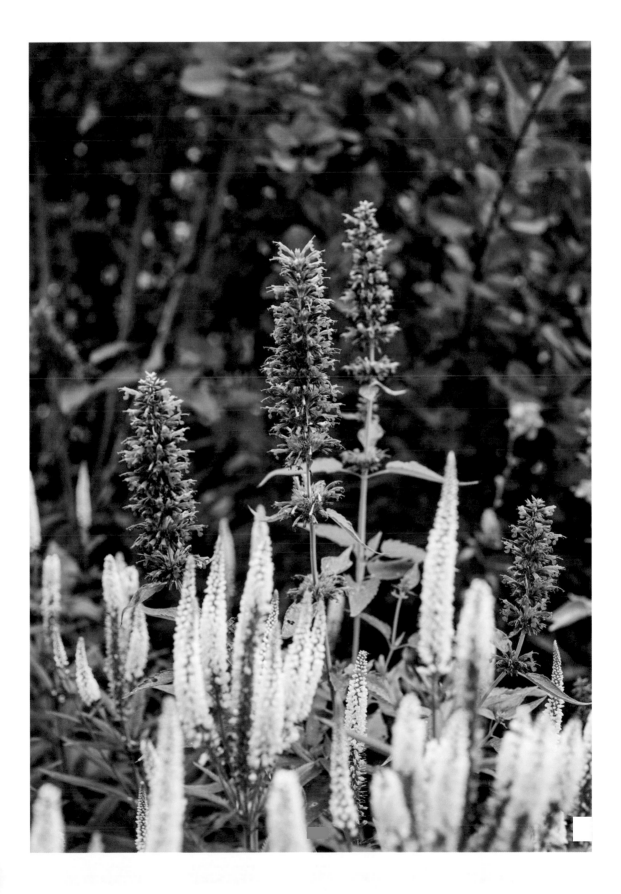

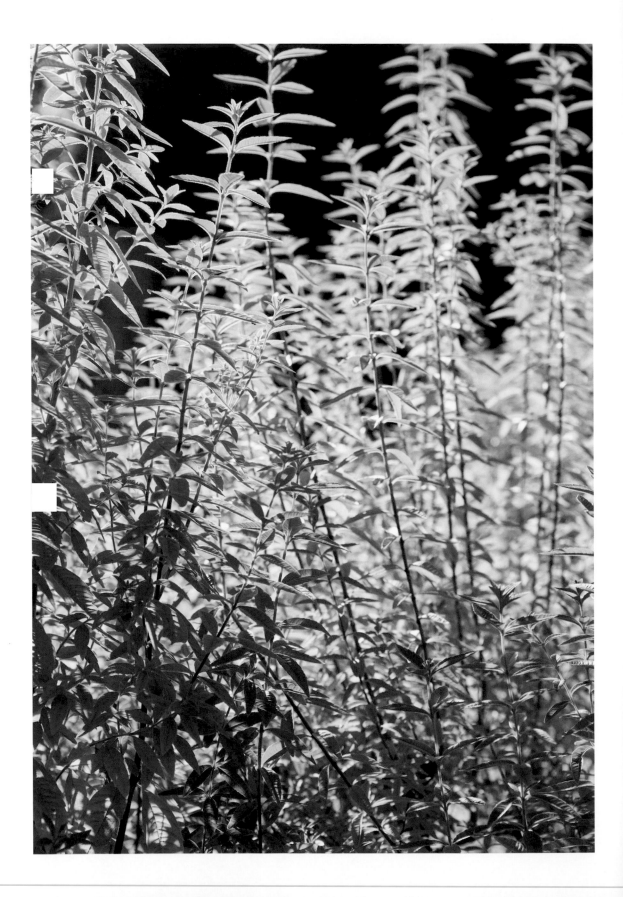

Aloysia citrodora

Lemon verbena

Zones 8–10 perennial, annual elsewhere

Full sun

Landscapes, culinary and medicinal gardens, containers

Lemony

Lemon verbena is a favorite and one of the most universally adored fragrant plants in the garden, with a strong and potent lemony scent. Its fragrance easily blends with other garden-grown natural scents. Lemon verbena has a place in all gardens.

Easily grown in containers, plants can be brought indoors to overwinter and then returned to the garden or a deck when spring arrives. Lemon verbena is pretty adaptable and can grow quite large in the landscape where it is perennial. Tiny white flowers appear in spring and early summer, but the plant does not always set seed. If you want to propagate lemon verbena, take cuttings.

The plant can get leggy if it's not pinched back regularly, so the more frequently you prune and harvest, the better. Use the foliage for fragrant iced tea and to make potpourri, hydrosols, oil infusions, lotions and salves, and candles. Lemon verbena is good in everything—except in arrangements, because it wilts quickly. If you do harvest for the vase, be sure to cut stems in the cool morning and place them in water immediately.

Antirrhinum spp.

Snapdragon, dragon flower

Zones 5–11 unreliable perennial, treat as an annual

Full sun to part shade

Cut flower gardens, culinary and medicinal gardens, containers

Honey, light, fruity, bubblegum

At one time, most garden snapdragons were scented. But as the plants have been hybridized by growers over the years, many of the more modern varieties are unscented—which is a shame. Snapdragons are beloved by most and are a staple in almost any garden.

Although snapdragons are technically perennials, you may find it less heartbreaking if you consider them annuals: that way, if they do stick around

lemon verbena

for more than a year, it is a bonus and not an expectation. Because of their ephemeral nature, snapdragons are best suited for dedicated cut flower gardens, edible and herb gardens, and containers. Flowers are ready to harvest when the lower third of the flower stem is in bloom. Harvest stems in the morning before the plant is in direct sunlight. Snapdragons are repeat bloomers, and as you harvest, more flowers appear. Be sure to store stems upright in the harvest bucket or the flower heads may begin to curve.

There are countless selections of snapdragons in every color, and we love them all, especially the flowers in the 'Azalea' series and traditional selections. They are easy to grow from seed. Look for unusual varieties such as the open-faced 'Chantilly' snapdragons for garden arrangements. Their florets tend to look a bit more like butterflies than dragon faces, but they are just as beloved.

Their unique blooms are beautiful in arrangements. Just a few are needed to add direction and movement. Snapdragons are also valued for their anti-inflammatory medicinal properties and can be combined with calendula in hand salves. Their scent can be a bit subtle on its own for perfumery, but it can be combined with more strongly scented plants to create a simple, gender-neutral fragrance.

Calamintha nepetoides

Lesser calamint	Landscapes, cut flower gardens
Zones 4–9	Minty, fresh
Full sun to part shade	

Calamint seems to bloom forever, with a flower show lasting from early summer through the first frost. A close cousin to culinary mint (*Mentha* spp.), calamint is a wonderful, minty, fresh-scented ground cover that is not invasive. It grows 12 to 18 inches tall and twice as wide, with a profusion of tiny, tubular, white or pale blue flowers produced on upright spikes. The clouds of tiny flowers attract bees, butterflies, and hummingbirds to the garden. This is an excellent plant for lining a pathway or at the front of a bed, where you can brush up against the foliage to release its fragrance. Plant it with roses, as the soft clouds of flowers make the roses' thorny bases easier on the eye.

Cut larger stems to add to flower arrangements as a frothy filler. We take inspiration from the garden and often combine calamint with roses in the vase.

'Chantilly Bronze' snapdragon

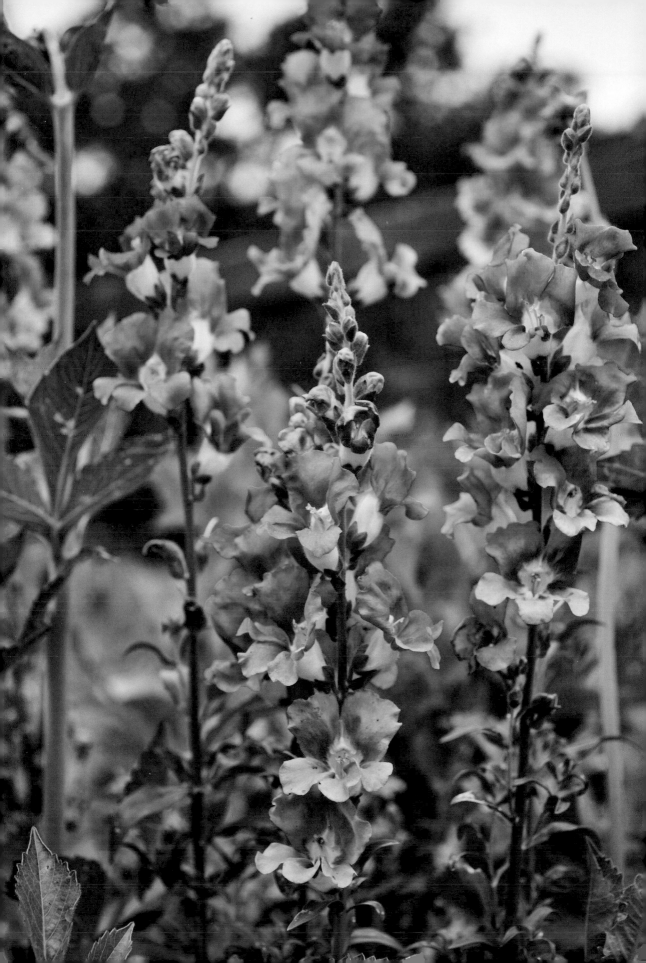

Flowers and leaves may stay fresh for a week or longer in the vase if kept out of direct sunlight. Favorites include the blue-flowered *C. nepeta* subsp. *nepeta* 'Blue Cloud' and white-flowered *C. nepeta* subsp. *glandulosa* 'White Cloud'.

Cosmos atrosanguineus

Chocolate cosmos	Landscapes, cut flower gardens
Zones 7–10 perennial, annual in zones 4–8	Chocolate
Full sun	

Chocolate cosmos is the embodiment of a chocolate flower, with deep maroon petals and a dark brown to black center—and it smells like chocolate! Utterly unique in the fragrant garden, the subtle chocolate aroma of this summer-bloomer makes it a must-have. The flowers' scent is most pronounced on hot, sunny summer days.

This tuberous perennial can grow in most gardens as a perennial or an annual. The chocolate-brown flowers attract butterflies and are good companions to most other flowers in the cut flower bed or landscape. Place chocolate cosmos at the front of a bed or in a container, where you can enjoy the chocolaty scent up close. Because deadheading encourages new growth, having easy access to these plants is important for keeping a continuing bloom of fresh, new flowers throughout the summer. The plant grows to 18 inches tall, with flowers on single stems of about 2 feet tall.

Most folks don't realize that chocolate cosmos grows from an underground tuber, similar to a dahlia. Like dahlia tubers, you can dig up chocolate cosmos tubers in the fall, divide them, overwinter them, and then replant them in the spring after frost if you live in a cold climate. *Cosmos atrosanguineus* is self-sterile, meaning it doesn't set seed, and it has traditionally been sold as a plant or as a tuber to plant in the garden. A relatively new cultivar, 'Black Magic', can be grown from seed, and its flowers produce viable seed; however, they are difficult to find and are quite expensive. We hope that chocolate cosmos 'Black Magic' seeds will become more widely available from seed companies. (See Resources on page 206 for more information.)

Chocolate cosmos pairs well with cut flowers in the dusky plant palette in both the garden and the vase. Sweet on their own, chocolate cosmos flowers are

chocolate cosmos

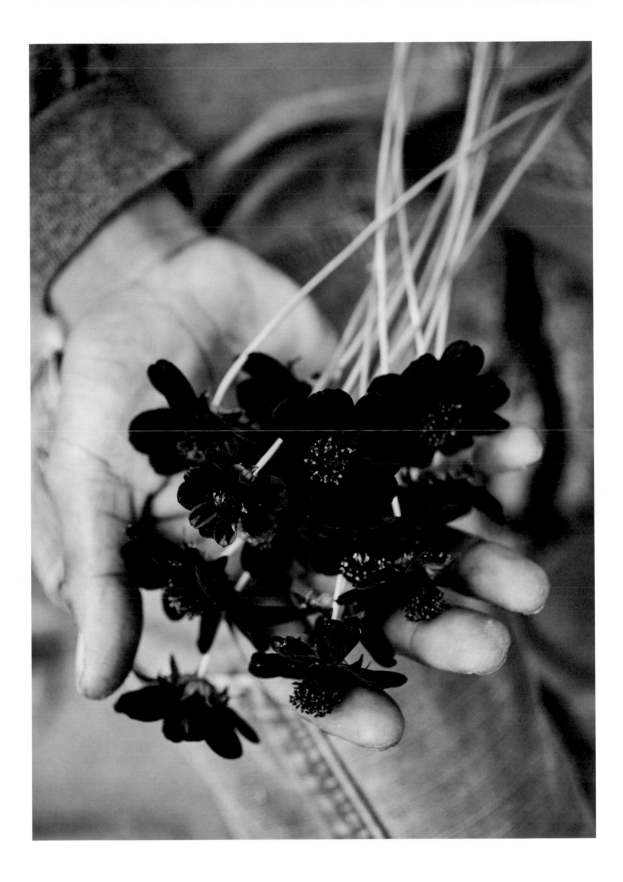

a great addition to arrangements. Stems are slender and delicate, so be careful with them as you work. Try bunching them together in small hand posies, versus using single stems, in larger arrangements so that they do not get lost. Chocolate cosmos can be quite expensive to purchase at a flower shop (if you can find them), so growing your own makes a lot of sense if you enjoy this flower. Their subtle fragrance is more fitting in a vase than for perfumery projects, but they can be blended with spice-scented blooms to create a unique scent.

Dianthus spp.

Pinks, carnation, sweet William
Zones 3–9
Full sun to part shade

Landscapes, cut flower gardens, culinary and medicinal gardens
Spicy-sweet, clove

Do not be afraid of pinks. Years ago, hybridizers did them dirty by breeding unscented, cheap, fluff-ball carnations instead of the lovely, clove-scented heirloom beauties that they should be. If you are one of the countless folks who turn up their noses at these flowers, it might be time to give them a second look.

Flower farmers and seed companies have done a lot to restore the reputation of this plant genus, and it is exciting to see all of the scented selections that are being reintroduced to gardeners. There are more than three hundred species of *Dianthus*, commonly known as pinks, carnations, or sweet Williams. All include some fragrant selections and all have edible flowers. There are so many to choose from for the garden! Open, single flowers and bicolored to long-stemmed, single and double flowers are available in violet, burgundy, and pastel pink. Favorites include the 'Chabaud' carnation series and the fragrant French heirloom 'Rose de Mai', which is valued for its uses in the kitchen as much as for the vase.

Harvest stems when a third to half of the blooms are open. The clove-scented flowers make a good and unexpected secondary flower in large arrangements and often last up to two weeks in the vase. Folks are often curious about these flowers in our arrangements, and they're surprised when we explain that the beautiful blooms are carnations! Their fragrance is really interesting in perfumery too. It is a good complementary scent that blends well with others.

Hedychium coronarium

Butterfly ginger

Zones 8–11

Part sun to part shade

Landscapes, cut flower gardens

Tropical honeysuckle

Along with frangipani (*Plumeria* spp.), butterfly ginger flowers produce an intoxicating fragrance often associated with Hawaii, but they can be grown on the mainland too. This plant is a must for the tropical-inspired fragrant garden.

Of all the fragrant gingers, butterfly ginger is the easiest growing tropical plant for nontropical gardens. The half-hardy perennial is as happy in a container as it is in a garden bed. Often grown as a die-back perennial in warmer states, this rhizomatous plant blooms from summer through fall. In zone 8 gardens, it will die back with the first frost, happily reappearing in early summer. This fast grower can reach heights of 6 to 7 feet in a single year; even if it dies back in winter, it will return with a force in spring. It needs regular, generous watering, though it will bloom and thrive with moderate amounts, making it a much more versatile plant than it appears.

Individual flowers resemble butterflies, hence its common name. A single pinecone-shaped spike on a thick, upright stalk produces clusters of creamy, pale yellow flowers with deep yellow throats. Individual flowers bloom for just a single day, starting from the bottom of the spike. Each day a new tier of flowers will bloom until eventually the last flowers at the top of the spike have their turn. After the flowers are done blooming, don't cut back the ginger's stalk to the ground. The large and beautiful foliage provides a tropical accent in a planting bed or container. In addition, the plant needs its foliage to collect and store energy for the following year's blooms. Note that butterfly ginger can be invasive in certain tropical parts of the world, including Hawaii, where it grows vigorously. If your garden is located in a tropical area, make sure to check your area's invasive plant species list before including it in your garden.

Butterfly ginger is a tall focal flower that demands attention in a vase. Harvest stalks when the plant is budded up and the bottom tier of flowers on the spike have just begun to open. Make sure that you harvest only as much stalk as you need for your vase, leaving some of the stalk and foliage in the garden. Each flower will open for about a day, but the stalk will keep blooming in the vase for multiple days. A cut stalk with open blooms at the top of the

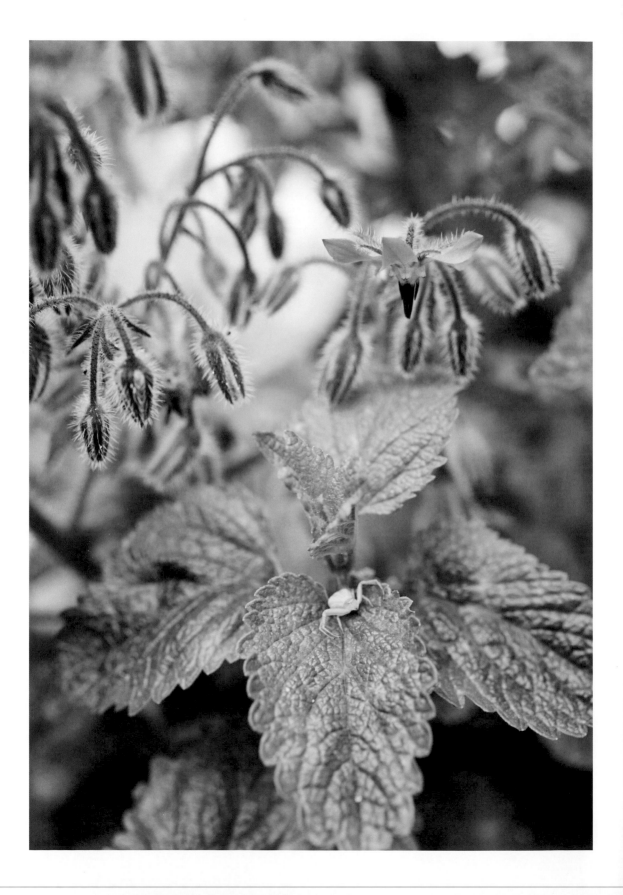

spike will last in a fragrant arrangement for only a day or two. To keep your arrangement looking fresh, remove the spent flowers daily.

Perfume is traditionally made with both the fragrant flowers and the plant's rhizomes, which are amazingly fragrant and edible. If you harvest the rhizome, remember that you are removing the entire plant from your garden. We typically harvest only flowers for perfumery projects unless we have more than enough rhizomes in the ground. The successive blooms make butterfly ginger flowers a good choice for tinctures and enfleurage that require small numbers of flowers and a longer period of time to infuse their scents.

Melissa officinalis

Lemon balm

Zones 4–9

Full sun to part shade

Landscapes, culinary and medicinal gardens, containers

Lemony, minty

It's funny that a plant known for its uplifting and carefree lemony aroma can cause so much stress in the garden! Fast-growing and invasive lemon balm is a good plant for the advanced gardener. It behaves similarly to mint and must be contained—or, better yet, given its own container.

Lemon balm refuses to stay put in the garden. New plants will pop up in other garden beds and along pathways. You can try to curtail the plant's wandering tendencies by pruning flowers before they go to seed or by pruning back the plant before the flowers emerge. Remove unwanted plants down to their roots. We set a weekly reminder to cut back and harvest lemon balm to keep it in check. This easy grower can be a good choice for difficult spots in your garden, such as a dry corner where no other plant will grow.

Lemon balm adds an informal touch to a garden arrangement, reminiscent of a backyard picnic. Use it as greenery or as a gestural touch in arrangements. Lemon balm mixes well with other lemon-scented plants. Harvest it for herbal teas and tea blends. Its strong citrus aroma persists even when the plant is dried.

lemon balm,
borage, and
garden spider

Mentha spp.

Mint

Zones 4–9

Full sun

Culinary and medicinal gardens, containers

Minty, spicy, herbal

Mint foliage is ideal for fragrant, garden-grown arrangements and is both beautiful and culinarily useful. Tall spikes of white flowers bloom in summer and add an artful touch to any garden or arrangement.

When you include mint in your garden, you will always have a constant supply. We rarely say this about a plant: keep mint out of your garden beds, unless you want a mint-filled landscape. Instead, plant it in a large container— the largest container you can find—because it will quickly outgrow smaller flower pots and will need to be repotted often. Even though it's a voracious grower, mint is a must. In a container, mint does best when it's harvested and fertilized often. Winter deciduous, it dies back following a frost, reemerging in the spring.

A variety of mint selections offer scents and textures that are fun to explore, including grapefruit mint (*M. citrata* 'Grapefuit'), lime mint (*M. citrata* 'Lime'), orange mint (*M.* × *piperita* f. *citrata* 'Orange'), pineapple mint (*M. suaveolens* 'Pineapple'), strawberry mint (*M.* × *piperita* 'Strawberry'), sweet pear mint (*M.* 'Sweet Pear'), and so many more. Peppermint (*M.* × *piperita*) and spearmint (*M. spicata*) plants also offer medicinal benefits, aiding in digestion and having a cooling effect on the body.

Harvest mint in the morning, and keep it bundled in a low vase with cool water, out of direct sunlight, until you are ready to use it. When harvesting large amounts for preservation, bind plants together with twine, give the cut ends a clean cut with your garden shears, and hang the bundles in a cool, dark place upside down. Dried stems can be used in wreath making or arrangements and are especially beautiful when the stems are dried with flowers intact. We blend multiple mint varieties in arrangements. Add single blooming sprigs of multiple varieties as secondary flowers or larger groups of stems as fragrant filler. Mint is a favorite to add to a fragrant kitchen wreath. We often harvest handfuls of mint just for simple kitchen arrangements to add to our cooking throughout the week. Combine mint with floral scents for oil infusions used for lip balms or hand salves for a cooling and refreshing effect.

'Chocolate' mint

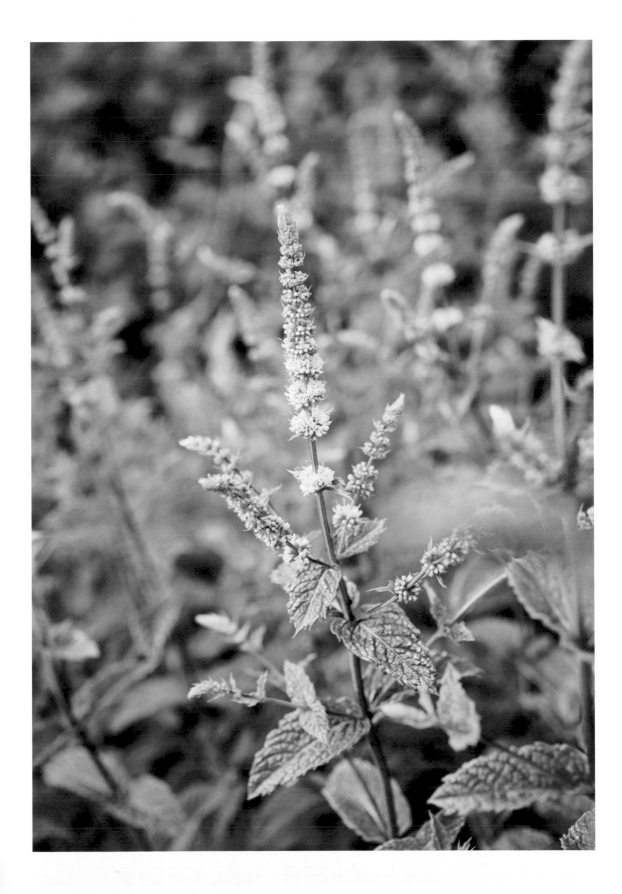

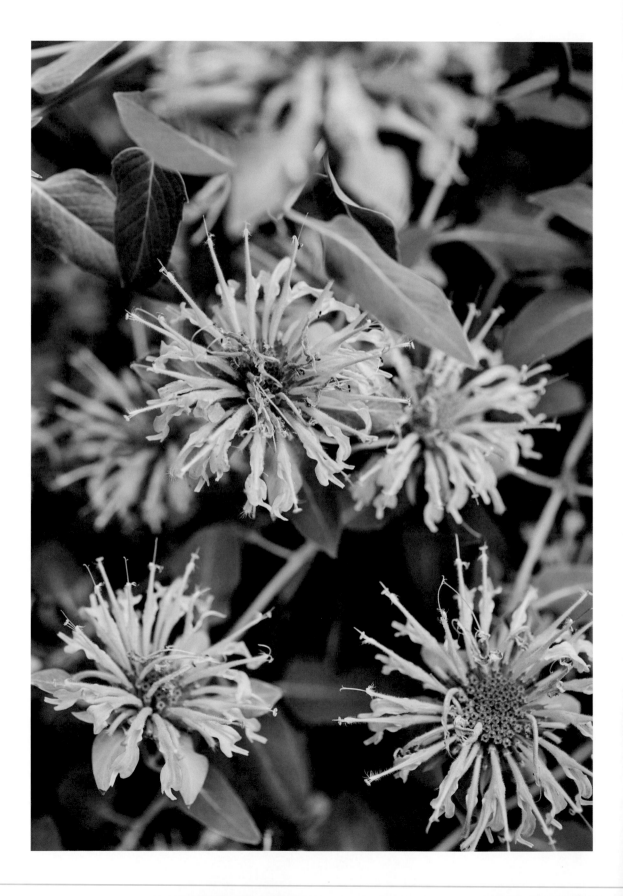

Monarda spp.

Bee balm

Zones 3–10

Full sun to part shade

Landscapes, culinary and medicinal gardens

Bergamot orange, sweetly bitter citrus

Each species of *Monarda* behaves differently in the garden. Bergamot (*M. didyma*), with red or bright pink flowers, aggressively spreads by runners and should be planted only in wide open spaces such as meadows, orchards, or on hillsides, where plants can spread freely. Lemon bee balm (*M. citrodora*), with purple flowers, is an annual that readily propagates and spreads by seed. Wild bergamot (*M. fistulosa*), with muted lavender flowers, is a clump-forming perennial that also spreads by runners but is not invasive. As bona fide bee, butterfly, and hummingbird magnets, bee balm blooms from summer until frost. Plants can grow 12 to 30 inches tall.

Bee balm's tiered clusters of tubular flowers are really beautiful and add a romantic touch to arrangements. The flowers hold their color in dried arrangements and wreaths, especially bergamot's bright pink, raspberry, magenta, and red blossoms. Although bee balm can easily overwhelm other flower fragrances, it adds a bright pop of floral and citrus notes when paired with roses and sage in fragrance blends.

Origanum vulgare

Oregano

Zones 4–10 perennial, annual elsewhere

Part sun to full sun

Landscapes, culinary and medicinal gardens, containers

Aromatic, camphorous

According to Roman legend, the goddess of love, Venus, gave the plant its scent "to remind mortals of her beauty." According to Ancient Greek mythology, Aphrodite, the goddess of love, created oregano as a symbol of joy. Oregano is at home in every garden. Its wonderful wandering habit makes it a natural for cascading over the edges of a raised bed, filling beds beside pathways, and

wild bergamot

mingling in meadow plantings. This adaptable, easy to grow herb is happiest in a sunny rock garden but will tolerate shade and wetter parts of the garden.

If you're planting oregano in a raised bed, place it along the edges (not in the middle) and let it cascade over the side (instead of letting it take over valuable bed space). One of our favorites is 'Dwarf Greek' oregano, which drapes beautifully. Oregano prefers full sun and will thrive where other plants fail in drier spots in the garden. Because oregano is a member of the mint family—notorious for its ability to spread—harvest it often to keep it in check.

Every part of the oregano—including the flowers, leaves, and stems—can and should be harvested and used. If it's a perennial plant where you live, harvest throughout late spring and summer and hang to dry and preserve. The plant will send up new stems for a fall harvest. For tea making and culinary uses, use sweeter selections such as 'Dwarf Greek', Italian oregano (*O. × majoricum*), or sweet marjoram (*O. majorana*). Because oregano is antimicrobial and antibacterial, it's an essential element in the fragrant medicinal garden.

Bees love oregano's beautiful purple and white blooms (depending upon variety), so it's a good idea to allow some plants to flower. The little blossoms are wonderful additions to summer arrangements and wreaths. Oregano flowers bring texture and fragrance to garden-grown arrangements as greenery, filler, and secondary flowers. Stems dry beautifully and can be used in wreaths. Add oregano to fragrant oil infusions and vinegar, or dry it to use in tea mixes. Our good friend Rose Loveall, owner at Morningsun Herb Farm, even suggests adding fresh stems to a hot bath at the onset of a cold.

Pelargonium spp.

Scented geranium

Zones 9–11 perennial, annual elsewhere

Full to part sun

Landscapes, cut flower gardens, culinary and medicinal gardens

Rose, fruity (including all citrus), nutty, minty, pungent

No herb or fragrant cut flower garden is complete without scented geranium. From foliage texture to fragrance, this plant offers outstanding diversity. Leaves range from smoothly rounded to finely cut and lacy, with colors ranging from gray to green. Seasonal blooms are typically white, apricot-toned, or pink. But it's really all about the scent—no other plant boasts as much aromatic variety!

'Mabel Grey' scented geranium

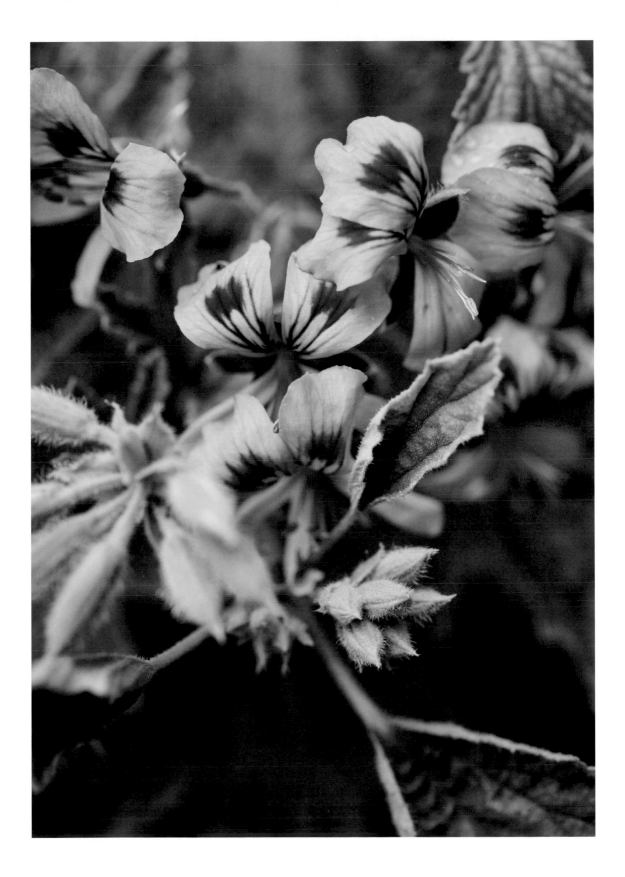

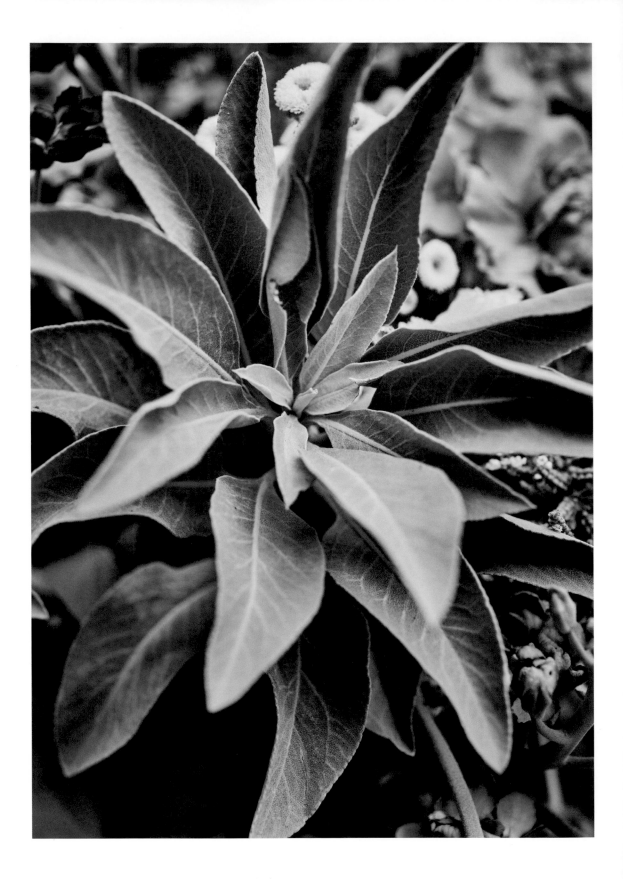

Scented geraniums can easily be grown in most gardens, either as perennials or annuals. In colder climates, you can plant them in containers so that they can be moved indoors for the winter. Whether they are planted in the garden or in a container, keep scented geraniums within easy reach, because their fragrance is released by gently rubbing their leaves.

There are more than 250 types of scented geranium, and most gardeners have a few favorites. They come in many shapes, colors, and fragrances. In the landscape, favorites include peppermint geranium (*P. tomentosum*) and its cultivar 'Chocolate' for their large, fuzzy leaves and sprawling growth habits. The low, dense foliage of 'Nutmeg' makes it a great choice for a scented pathway, and no cut flower or herb garden should be without 'Mabel Grey' and 'Skeleton Rose'. *Pelargonium graveolens* 'Colocho' is a favorite for its unusual twisted leaves as well as its citrus floral aroma.

Harvest stems liberally to create fragrant foliage bases, and use the flowering stems as gestural elements in arrangements. Scented geranium oil has mood-enhancing and uplifting medicinal qualities. Essential oils are typically made from the more famous herbaceous and rose-scented geraniums. Citrus-scented geraniums offer unusual, hard-to-find fragrances. Making a fragrant infusion with citrus-scented geraniums is a great way to get citrus fragrance from a non-citrus plant—after all, not everyone can grow lemons, but we all can grow lemon-scented geraniums. Lemon-scented geraniums also pair well with roses and other scented flowers and add a touch of citrus to any garden arrangement. Heat activates scented geraniums' fragrance, so it is no surprise that adding a leaf or two to a hot cup of tea or adding a single stem to a hot bath can transform the experience.

Salvia apiana

White sage, bee sage
Zones 8–10
Full sun

Landscapes, culinary and medicinal gardens
Herbaceous, clean, dry

White sage has a unique fragrance. It is nearly impossible to walk by the plant and not run your hands through the silver-white foliage, activating its scent. This drought-tolerant salvia likes a dry summer and is not suitable for gardens with humid, wet summers. It pairs beautifully with other flowering

white sage

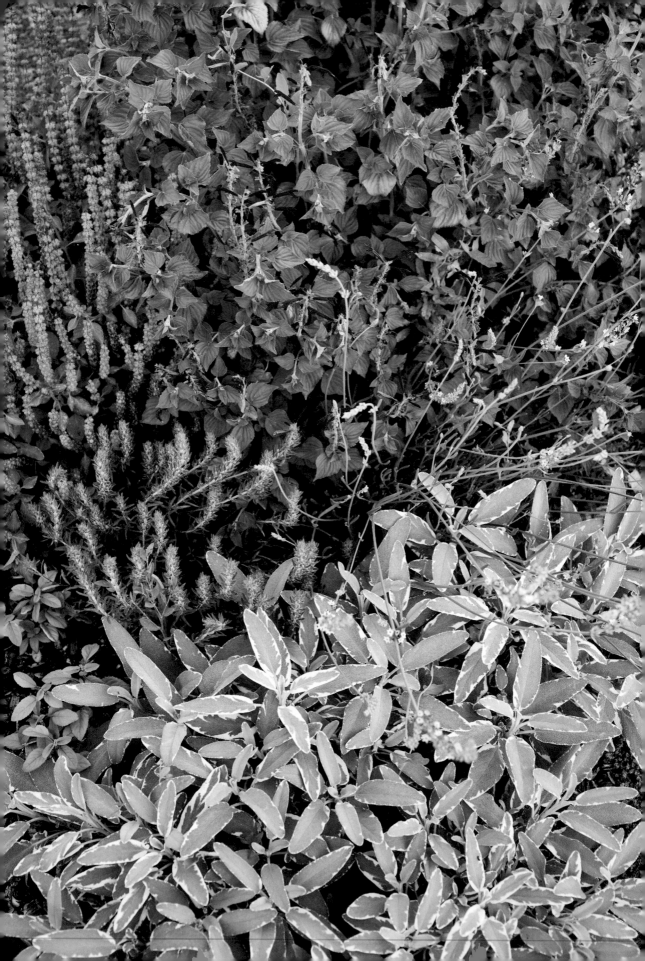

mediterranean plants, grasses, and succulents. Include it in meadow plantings, gravel gardens, or any bee-friendly garden. *Apiana* is Latin for "belonging to bees"—bee sage is bee heaven!

This plant's scent is intoxicating. To release it, you can burn or rub the foliage or flowers or distill their essences. Its silver-white foliage is beautiful in an arrangement, especially when the white flower spikes are in bloom in the summer. It is a key ingredient in our medicinal-based arrangements. Mix it with sprigs of rosemary, thyme, blooming oregano, bee balm, Cleveland sage, or any pleasantly scented medicinal plant. After enjoying the fresh arrangement for about a week, simply remove the stems from water, trim off the water-decayed parts, and bind the stems with twine. Hang them upside down to dry in a cool, dark place. When the plants are dry in about two weeks, they can be used for fragrant projects. Fresh stems and foliage are wonderful in infusions and distillations.

Salvia elegans

Pineapple sage	Landscapes, culinary and medicinal gardens, containers
Zones 8–11	
Full sun	Pineapple, sweet, fruity, hints of mint and spice

Salvia elegans is easy to grow, has a long bloom cycle, and is happy to grow in dry conditions, though it also thrives with regular water. Its dramatic spikes of tubular scarlet flowers are hummingbird favorites. These plants can grow quite large, to 5 feet tall and 3 feet wide, and are best located at the back of the border. Smaller selections are more manageable for dedicated herb or edible planting beds. Tangerine sage (*S. elegans* 'Tangerine') is 3 feet tall and wide and makes a wonderful flowering backdrop plant for the herb bed. 'Honey Melon' is a smaller selection, at 2 feet tall and wide, that can be planted in the middle to front section of an herb bed, where its constant profuse and fruit-scented flowers can be appreciated. Smaller yet is 'Golden Delicious', at 12 to 24 inches tall and 30 inches wide, with chartreuse foliage. It makes a good container plant.

Pineapple sage is beautiful in a wildflower arrangement, but flowers do not typically have a long vase life. The sweet and spicy scented foliage and flowers are wonderful additions to citrus or floral scents in infusions to make salves and balms.

tulsi basil, 'Tangerine' sage, 'Edelweiss' lavender, 'Tricolor' sage

Salvia officinalis

Sage, culinary sage

Zones 5-8, annual elsewhere

Full sun

Landscapes, culinary and medicinal gardens, containers

Minty, camphorous, slightly peppery, earthy

In the garden, *Salvia officinalis* has a tidy mounding habit. It requires little to no maintenance and emits a classic earthy aroma that smells like home. It may not be a reliable bloomer, but that's OK, because this sage is all about the plump and oval, fragrant leaves.

Available in green, purple, and variegated leaf colors, culinary sage is an evergreen perennial subshrub in its primary hardiness zones. It can be grown as an annual or overwintered indoors in colder areas. Compact and woody stemmed, culinary sage typically grows 12 to 24 inches tall and is both drought tolerant and deer resistant. This plant can thrive with neglect and often dies when it is pampered. Its fuzzy leaves add texture to a container, planting bed border, or rock garden, and its low, cascading growth habit makes it a fantastic choice for an edging plant in a raised bed, in herb and culinary garden beds, or along a pathway.

Harvest larger stems for use in arrangements, garlands, and kitchen wreaths. Dried sage has a stronger flavor than fresh, so we collect the dried leaves to include in garlands and wreaths and to make winter teas. The muted colors of culinary sage are pretty in arrangements and add a nice, spicy aroma that blends well with floral scents. Although its fragrance is pleasant, it is not one that would typically be worn as perfume and is better enjoyed in candles, hydrosols, and dried wreaths.

Sideritis cypria

Cyprus ironwort, mountain tea

Zones 7–11

Full sun

Landscapes, culinary and medicinal gardens

Minty, oregano

With beautiful, soft, velvety silver leaves, Cyprus ironwort is a favorite fragrant, low-growing plant for the dry garden. In its native Cyprus, it is rare

Cyprus ironwort in bloom

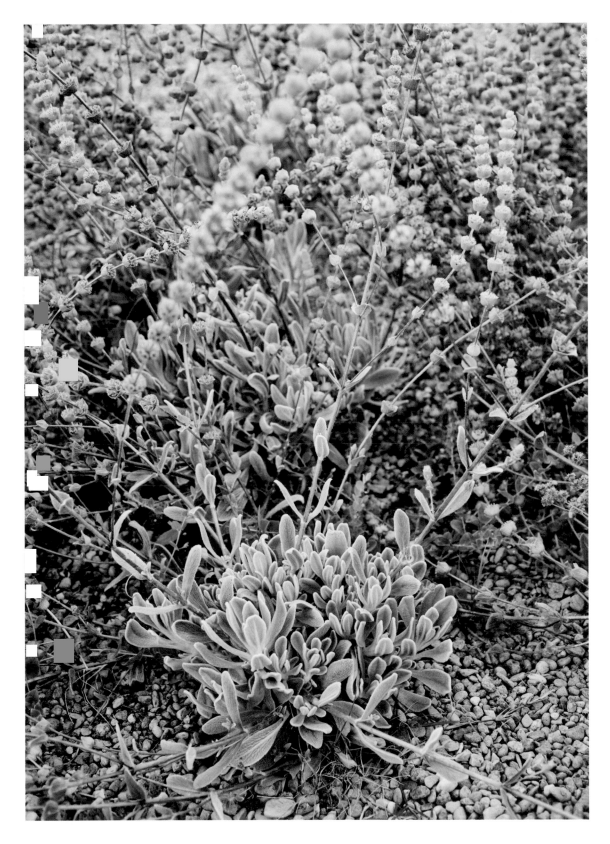

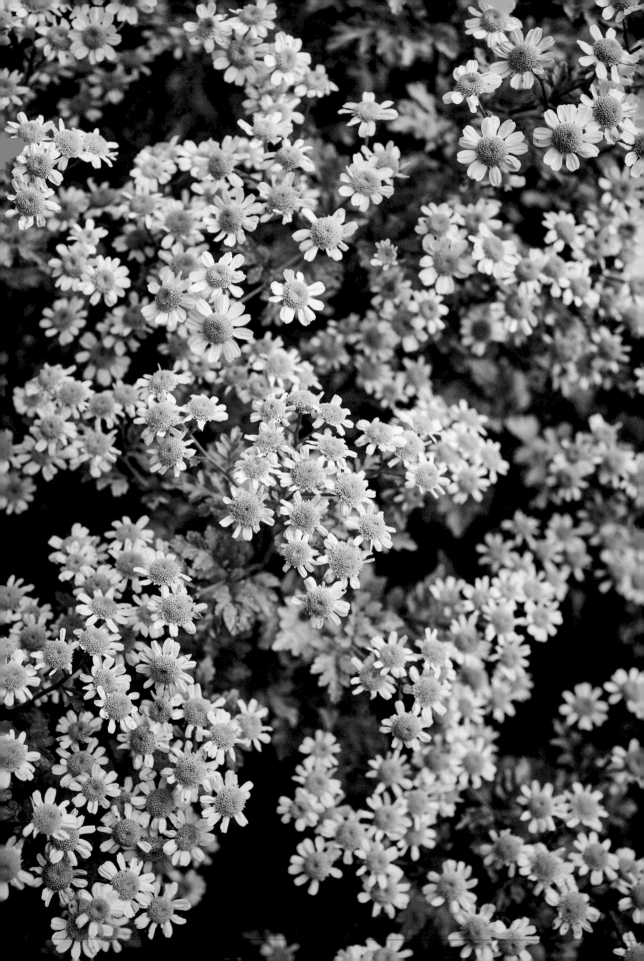

and considered endangered, but where it is hardy in North America, it is at home in a dry rock or gravel garden. With minty, oregano-scented leaves, Cyprus ironwort is beloved as a tea ingredient.

The fragrant silver foliage base of the plant has a nice mounding habit and grows to about 2 feet tall, which makes it an excellent choice for edging a bed or pathway. Just one look at the plant will tell you that it is a close relative of lamb's ears (*Stachys* spp.); in fact, both are in the same plant family. When designing a low-water garden, you can use Cyprus ironwort instead of lamb's ears in an area that receives more water—think of it as a fragrant alternative. You can also add it alongside succulents and fescues (grasses) to add a fragrant touch, or plant it with fragrant, dry-loving lavender, rosemary, white sage, and yarrow.

In the summer, Cyprus ironwort puts on a show with tall, wiry stems of green flowers, which are actually cup-shaped calyces. These are a bit buttonlike in appearance and start off chartreuse, fading to silver during summer's hot days. The unusual flowers are fantastic in dried arrangements and wreaths and add a gestural touch to fresh arrangements. Harvest its leaves year-round as you need them for tea and perfumery projects. Both the leaves and flowers can be used in distillations for a refreshing hydrosol.

Tanacetum parthenium

Feverfew	Landscapes, cut flower gardens, culinary and medicinal gardens, containers
Zones 5–10	
Full sun	
	Medicinal, strong, bitter

Traditionally included in medicinal gardens, feverfew has bright, cheery, daisylike flowers that belong in the cut flower garden as well. Because their strong scent is not for everyone and actually deters bees, it is a good plant to include along a high-traffic pathway where you may want to discourage the stinging insects. By the same token, avoid planting feverfew near fruit trees or fruiting shrubs that need bees for pollination.

Feverfew is an easily grown perennial or annual herb that has traditionally been used to treat a variety of conditions, including migraine headaches, arthritis, and, as its name implies, fevers. Feverfew flowers resemble those

golden feverfew   of German chamomile (*Matricaria chamomilla*), which is in the same plant family, and the two plants are sometimes confused. You can smell the flowers to distinguish between the two. Feverfew flowers have a strong, bitter, and medicinal scent, unlike the mellow chamomile aroma. Feverfew also has a more vertical growth habit than the famous tea herb, reaching 24 inches tall, with lacy foliage and long, thin stems.

You can plant feverfew from seed. Sprinkle them throughout dedicated cut flower and herb garden beds in spring, but do not cover the seeds because they need sunlight to germinate. Feverfew prefers full sun but will grow in partial shade with less flowering. It is relatively carefree and can thrive in poor soils with moderate water. It reseeds easily and will spread prolifically throughout the garden if not controlled. Deadhead spent flowers to control unwanted self-seeding. If a new plant appears where it is not welcome, simply dig it up and plant it elsewhere—feverfew is easily transplanted.

Flowering stems are a welcome addition to summer garden arrangements as a filler or secondary flower. Feverfew's anti-inflammatory qualities make it a great ingredient for fragrant oils and salves when combined with more floral- or herbaceous-scented plants. Its bitter, medicinal scent is pleasing for some but not for everyone.

Thymus spp.

Thyme	Landscapes, culinary and medicinal gardens, containers
Zones 3b–11	
Full sun	Herbaceous, minty

Strolling along a path lined with fragrant thyme is one of the great pleasures of being in the garden. A member of the mint family and a relative of oregano, thyme is an evergreen, fragrant herb that is bountiful in its culinary, medicinal, and ornamental uses in the garden. Common thyme, *T. vulgaris*, is used as a culinary herb. The plant's fragrance can vary depending on the species or cultivar. Look for caraway thyme (*T. herba-barona*), lavender-scented thyme (*T. thracicus*), lemon thyme (*T. citriodorus*), and orange-scented thyme (such as *T. vulgaris* 'Orange Balsam'). Creeping thyme (*T. serpyllum*) is a favorite ground cover that releases its fragrance when you step on it!

Thyme should be harvested frequently in big bundles or it will begin to look scruffy in the garden. Use it to flavor fragrant vinegar infusions and herbal salves and oils, or dry and preserve it to add to fragrant tea blends and herb garlands and wreaths.

Viola odorata

Sweet violet

Zones 4–10a

Part shade to shade

Landscapes, culinary and medicinal gardens, containers

Berrylike, sweet

The genus *Viola* comprises a large group of cheerful, edible, and often fragrant plants. The most fragrant species in the genus is *V. odorata*. The petal colors of sweet violet vary from deep violet to white. Its heart-shaped foliage may explain why it was once believed to have healing properties that provided comfort to those suffering from heartache.

Favorite cultivars include the deep purple flowers of *V. odorata* 'Königin Charlotte' (Queen Charlotte) and lavender flowers of *V.* 'Duchesse de Parme', both among the most fragrant cultivars. Sweet violets are a must for shadier parts of the fragrant garden. Plant them along the edges of garden beds or use them as a ground cover and along pathways, where you can appreciate these petite and beautifully scented plants. *Viola odorata* is also a wonderful plant for containers.

Harvest flowers in abundance throughout the spring to extend the blooming season. The more you harvest, the more this plant will bloom. Use fresh flowers immediately or put them on a drying rack and let the blooms air-dry (which typically takes about forty-eight hours). The small and delicate flowers will get lost in larger arrangements. Harvest a few stems for an intimate bedside arrangement or to make simple nosegays, or take inspiration from Alethea's grandmother, who would pin a few to her blouse with a broach. Use the flowers in infusions and tinctures for perfumery projects.

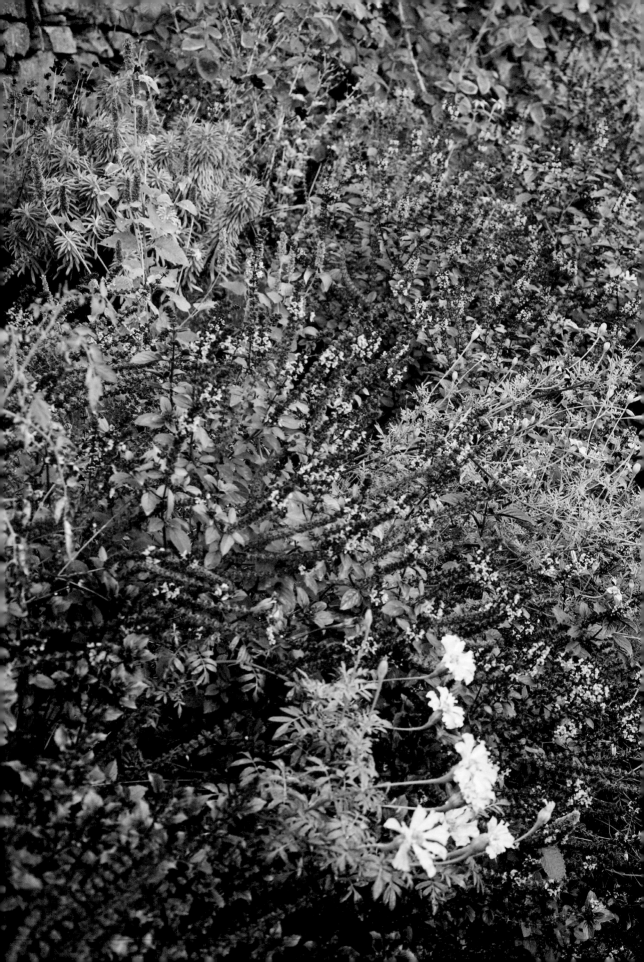

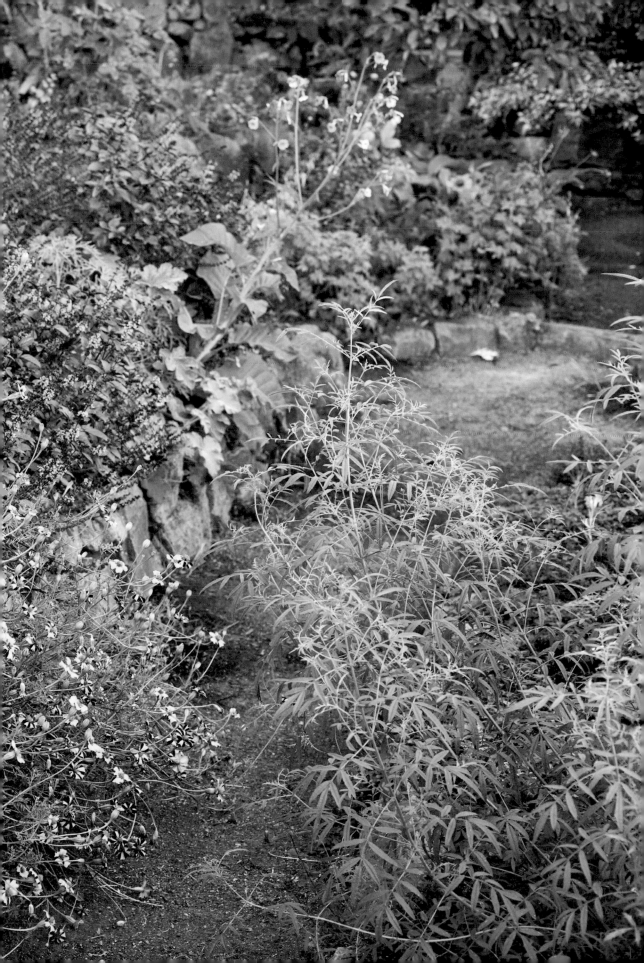

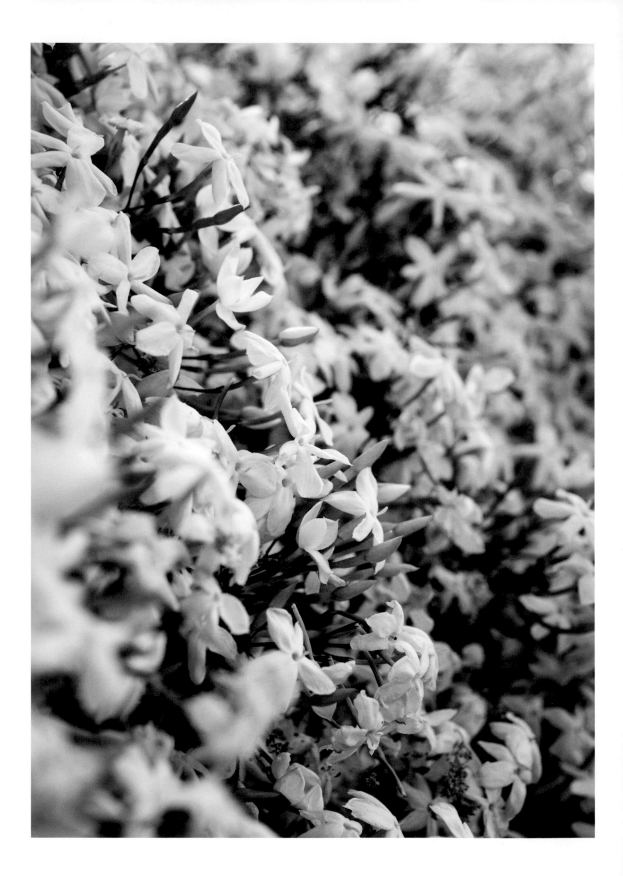

VINES

Jasminum spp. and others

Jasmine
Zones 6–12 (selection dependent)
Full sun to part shade

Landscapes, cut flower gardens, culinary and medicinal gardens
Rich, honey-sweet

The name *jasmine* is derived from a Persian word that means "gift from God" or "fragrant flower." This genus produces some of the most sacred and fragrant flowers in the world. The large genus of flowering vines and shrubs includes about 200 different species. The common name "jasmine" is shared by many fragrant-flowered shrubs and vines from other genera as well, including two favorites—star jasmine (*Trachelospermum jasminoides*) and Madagascar jasmine (*Stephanotis floribunda*). Volumes of books could be written about this plant.

Before you include jasmine to your garden, you need to know your growing conditions and choose a selection that can thrive there. Once you plant jasmine, there is no going back—it immediately becomes an integral part of the fragrant garden. Depending on an individual plant's growth habit (either shrub or vine), jasmine should be placed near a pathway or window, where you can readily enjoy its scent. In either form, jasmine adds a beautiful, fragrant texture to the garden's scent palette that accentuates all other fragrances in the very best way. When grown on an arbor or trellis, vining varieties can be focal points and anchors. If a blank garden fence needs covering, vining jasmine will quickly do the job. For gardens in colder climates, many varieties can be grown in containers and overwintered indoors, and some varieties are valued as fragrant houseplants.

Make sure you have easy access to the plant so that you can harvest flowers to enjoy inside, where their pervasive fragrance will immediately let everyone know that jasmine is in the room. To prolong the flowers' vase life, harvest long stems in the morning when flowers are halfway to a third of the way open, untwining the stems as you harvest. Because the stems can get

pink jasmine

visually lost in larger arrangements, create a small hand posy before placing them in the vase. Long stems are beautiful spilling out of a vase, hanging from a mantel, or spreading across a table. To celebrate jasmine's amazing fragrance while it is in bloom, capture and preserve the flowers' scent in an infusion or distillation, or dry the blossoms for other uses.

Each of these favorite jasmines has a quality that is unique and brings value to any fragrant garden.

JASMINUM SPP.

Arabian jasmine (*J. sambac*): Zones 9–11 (the basis for jasmine tea)

Pink jasmine (*J. polyanthum*): Zones 8–11

Royal jasmine (*J. grandiflorum*): Zones 8–10 (French perfume jasmine, *J. grandiflorum* 'Flora Plena', is grown in France for perfumery)

Common jasmine (*J. officinale*): Zones 7–10

Winter jasmine (*J. nudiflorum*): Zones 6–10

OTHER GENERA

Madagascar jasmine (*Stephanotis floribunda*): Zone 12 (can be grown as a houseplant)

Night-blooming jasmine (*Cestrum nocturnum*): Zones 8–11

Star jasmine (*Trachelospermum jasminoides*): Zones 8–10

Lonicera spp.

Honeysuckle

Zones 4–11

Full sun to part shade

Landscapes, cut flower gardens

Strongly honey-sweet, vanilla, floral

With flowers that provide fragrance on happy, hot summer days, honeysuckle is a rambunctious flowering vine that needs space to climb and ramble. Give it a sturdy fence or an arbor on the borders or the outer edges of the garden. Honeysuckle provides a great solution for covering up an unsightly chain-link fence. This vining plant will devour the fence, covering it with butterfly-shaped perfumed blooms. Winter-deciduous honeysuckle represents all things wild in the garden, in the very best way.

Harvest honeysuckle flowers generously for arrangements and perfumery. The flowers are sweetly fragrant and contain a drop of "honey" (nectar) that you can suck from the tip of the pulled flower. Easy to mix with other flowers in a vase, honeysuckle's flowers, long vines, and branches are great focal parts. Individual stems can be added as a gestural touch, draping out of the vase. It can be laborious to preserve honeysuckle's scent, because it requires that you pull each open blossom from the vine individually to fill a container of carrier oil or alcohol. Then blooms must be switched out daily because the petals rot quickly and will spoil an infusion. It is best to distill a large harvest of the blooms all at once (although it is still a laborious process).

Passiflora spp.

Passion flower, passion vine	Landscapes, cut flower gardens, culinary and medicinal gardens
Zones 5–9	
Full sun to part shade	Tropical, vanilla, clove, spicy

The flowers of this vining perennial are highly decorative, and most are tropically fragrant. Don't be fooled by the delicate appearance of this vine, because passion flower is a vigorous plant that can take over a fence, a wall, or even a house! Passion flower refuses to be ignored in the garden. It must be actively reined in and cut back heavily in the winter to keep its growth in check. This is great news if you planted passion flower with a dual purpose in mind—for its fragrance, plus to harvest for teas, flowers arrangements, perfumery projects, and fruit.

Many passion flowers are host plants for butterflies and are moderately drought tolerant, though they thrive with plenty of water. Not all selections are fragrant, so do your homework before you include the plant in your garden. Favorites include the tropical-spicy fragrances of *P. phoenicea* 'Ruby Glow' and cultivars 'Purple Tiger' and 'Incense', the latter of which is especially root-hardy and a good choice for gardens in colder areas.

Before cutting vines for arrangements, unwind and separate individual stems so that you can take a long stem cutting for the vase. To prevent the long stems from dehydrating and going limp, condition them in a tall bucket of lukewarm water, preferably overnight, before using them in arrangements. The fragrant flowers are very delicate, so they are best added last. If you hope to harvest passion fruit, a happy passion vine can produce plenty, even if you harvest some vines for the vase and perfume projects. This vine is a major producer, so go for it and harvest at all stages of the plant's production. Add passion flowers to tropical-inspired infusions or mix them with citrus and floral scents in garden blends.

Wisteria spp.

Wisteria	Landscapes, cut flower gardens
Zones 4–9	Very sweet and floral, sometimes musky
Full sun to part shade	

Beloved by many, wisteria is one of the earliest bloomers of the winter-deciduous fragrant vines. This climber's sweet-smelling flower clusters emerge in the final days of winter, signaling spring's approaching arrival. Because a mature wisteria can be quite large, with vines of 20 to 30 feet long, it can destroy all but the sturdiest fences because of its weight. Many gardeners choose to grow this rambunctious vine on their home's façade or on a pergola, where it serves as a focal plant in the garden. The vine's light purple, blue, or pink flowers grow in large, drooping clusters (racemes).

Two species of wisteria are commonly grown in the United States: Japanese wisteria (*W. floribunda*) and Chinese wisteria (*W. sinensis*). Both are aggressive growers and are considered invasive in many parts of the country. American wisteria (*W. frutescens*) is a good noninvasive choice for the fragrant garden. Native to the Eastern United States, it is a less aggressive, slower growing vine with short but fragrant flower clusters. Flowers appear only on new growth, so keep that in mind as you prune.

Wisteria's ephemeral beauty, when its flowers first emerge, is hard to beat, and the sweet and fruity fragrance of its blossoms signals the arrival of the magical days of spring. As the flowers age, their sweet aroma grows more intense. As the mature, large vines abundantly bloom, many find that the aroma can be sickly sweet or cloying. This is a good time to harvest them for the vase and for perfumery projects.

'Aunt Dee' wisteria

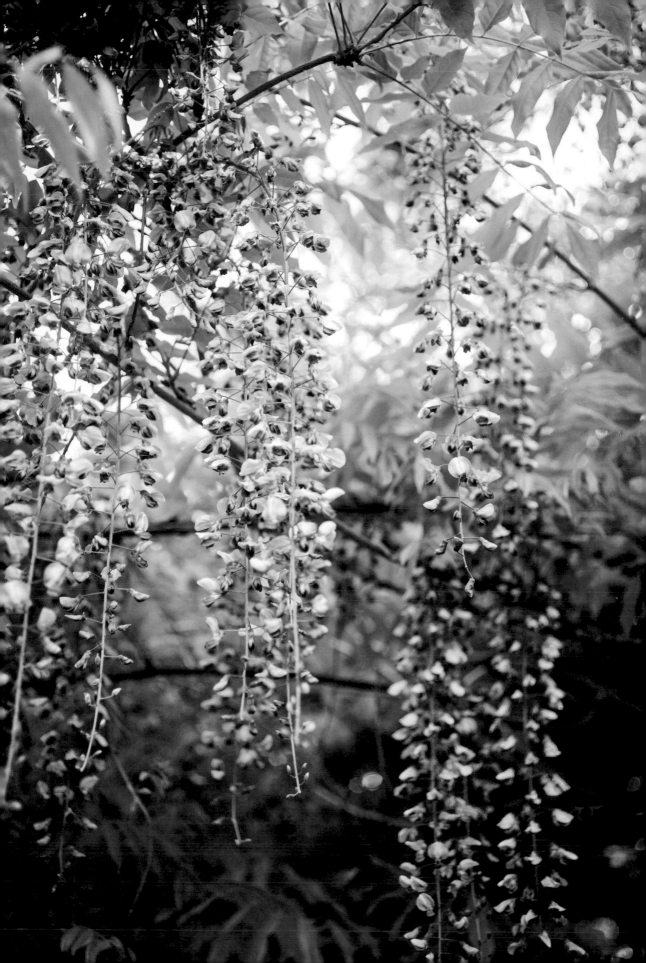

When harvesting for the vase, choose stems with both open and unopen flower heads to lengthen their vase life. When composing an arrangement, add wisteria to the vase last, because the flowering vines can be very tender. In an arrangement, use wisteria as a draping, vining component to create a romantic, Bohemian effect. In a tall arrangement, wisteria spills out of the vase and can be quite stunning. When using wisteria with other early spring–blooming flowers in an arrangement, keep fragrance in mind and avoid including other strong-scented blooms such as paperwhites. The scents tend to clash instead of complementing one another.

Save your wisteria prunings to create beautiful wreath bases. Directly after pruning, while stems are still pliable, form the wreath's shape and connect the ends with florist's wire. The wreath base can be dried and stored or used right away.

Most commercially available wisteria-scented perfumes and products don't smell like the plant, as perfumers typically use a synthetic version of the scent. But you can harvest and preserve your fresh wisteria immediately. Use infusion and distillation techniques to create a single scent, or blend wisteria with other, less intense, scents. Embrace the moment and create a multifloral explosion blend.

BULBS, CORMS, RHIZOMES & TUBERS

Agave amica

Tuberose

Zones 9–11 perennial, annual
elsewhere

Full sun to part shade

Landscapes, cut flower gardens

Jasmine, gardenia, frangipani

A tropical plant for a nontropical garden, the tuberose is not for the fragrant faint of heart. Some say its complex fragrance resembles that of diaper cream, but in a really good way. Others compare it to gardenia, with hints of jasmine and buttered popcorn.

A tropical/subtropical bulb, tuberose is at home in the dedicated cut flower garden. It prefers to grow in areas where the soil does not freeze. If you are growing it in colder areas, you can treat it as an annual bulb, as you would a dahlia. Remove its tubers in the fall, store them in a dry and cool space for the winter, and replant them in the spring.

Tuberose's cream-colored, waxy flowers appear on a single, spire-shaped stem. They blend well with other midlevel cut flowers in the front or middle sections in the garden bed, where the blooms are not visually overpowered by taller plants. Once it is finished blooming, the tuberose's grasslike foliage is unremarkable, so it's best to include it in a mixed-flower planting, where the foliage can blend in. Snails and slugs like the fleshy bulb leaves that emerge from the ground in spring, so keep an eye out for these pests to protect the bulb's new growth.

It can be difficult to convince tuberose flower buds to open if you purchase a budded spike at a flower shop instead of growing the plant yourself. Harvest your homegrown flowers when half of the individual flowers on the stem are already open, in the morning before the plant is exposed to direct sunlight. A few stems go a long way in an arrangement: tuberose can be overpowering if you use too many along with other flowers. A single stem can be used as the pointer in an asymmetrical arrangement, and adding a vase with a single stem or two by the bedside is a lovely way to experience tuberose's fragrance. When used sparingly, tuberose combines with many scents, especially woody and musky fragrances. Harvest individual flower heads for flower tinctures and enfleurage projects. Most commercially available tuberose-scented products are synthetic because the plant's essential oil is very expensive.

Convallaria majalis

Lily of the valley	Landscapes, cut flower gardens
Zones 2–9	Sweet, fresh, jasmine
Part shade to full shade	

Where the nodding, bell-shaped, white flowers of lily of the valley line a wild woodland pathway in spring, they create a favorite spring fragrance moment. The plant's fragile appearance contrasts with its flowers' strong fragrance, which is valued everywhere. Lily of the valley is an old-fashioned scent that we look forward to every year. It is dainty, strong, beautiful, and precious, and there is nothing quite like it in the shade garden.

In shady woodland plantings, lily of the valley grows by rhizomes and easily naturalizes (the bulbs multiply underground) throughout the landscape where it grows. It blooms best after a hard, cold winter and does not thrive in hot, humid climates. It is at its best when grown as a shaded ground cover with room to roam. As the rhizomes naturalize and multiply, they grow closer together, forming a dense mat. Deer and rabbit resistant, all parts of this plant are toxic if ingested.

Lily of the valley is a romantic flower, and it's also a symbol of good luck. It's no surprise that its tiny flowering stems are favorites for nosegays, boutonnieres, and for tucking into bridal bouquets. Combine it with other small blooms such as daphnes, violets, grape hyacinths (*Muscari* spp.), and fritillaries (*Fritillaria* spp.) in small, delicate arrangements. Its tiny flowers will get lost in larger arrangements.

Lily of the valley is an essential part of many floral scent blends. Because it's nearly impossible to extract essential oil from these little flowers, and doing so requires copious amounts of blooms, commercially available perfumes often use a synthetic scent. We use lily of the valley enfleurage and flower tinctures for our garden-based perfumery projects.

Freesia spp.

Freesia

Zones 9–10 perennial, annual bulb elsewhere

Full sun to part shade

Landscapes, cut flower gardens, containers

Sweet, floral tea with honey and lemon

With a scent reminiscent of a cup of floral tea with a touch of citrus, freesia's flowers are familiar yet difficult to describe. There is nothing else quite like it. Freesia's skinny stems emerge in spring with flowers that uniquely grow horizontally. Newer hybrids are not as fragrant as the species but are available in many colors in both single and double blooms. The bicolor varieties are also real stunners.

In the garden, freesias tend to be left alone by deer and are not fussy when it comes to soil type. In colder climates, growing freesia in containers is a good choice because their corms (underground storage organs) can be easily removed and stored to replant the following year. Make sure to choose a tall container, however, because freesias have long tap roots and need space. This South African native prefers dry summers and mediterranean climates. If your garden experiences summer rain, this is another reason to plant freesias in containers, because you can adjust the summer watering to enable the corms to go dormant before removing them to store for the following year.

The long, sword-shaped leaves need to continue to grow and collect nutrients to strengthen the corm for the following year's growth. Allow the foliage to die back before removing it. Freesia can be easily forced in vases indoors. In summer-dry climates where freesias can happily live outdoors, add them to fragrant meadow plantings, along a fragrant pathway, and in dedicated cut flower beds. If you garden in a mediterranean climate and can find false freesia (*F. laxa* 'Alba'), it is a favorite that has the best freesia fragrance. When happy, it easily naturalizes in the landscape.

Freesia provides a pretty silhouette in arrangements and has a long vase life. Harvest stems when a quarter to a third of the flowers are open, as buds will continue to bloom in the vase. It is easy to remove spent flower heads in an arrangement to keep it looking fresh for a week or two. In perfumery, freesias blend well with other flowers. Try making a flower tincture with herbaceous scented plants or an infusion with floral scented ones.

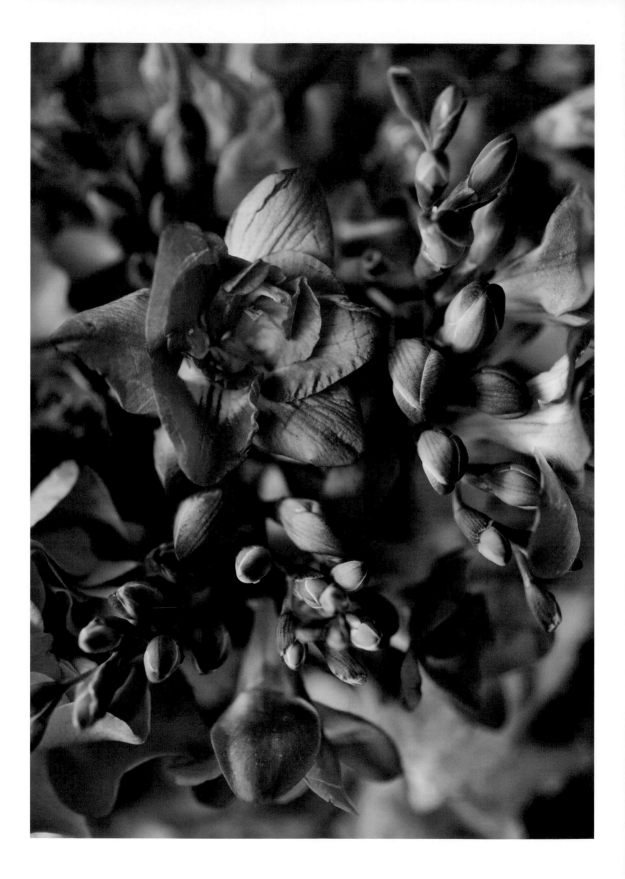

Hyacinthus spp.

Hyacinth
Zones 4–8, treat as an annual bulb
Full sun to part shade

Landscapes, cut flower gardens, containers
Pungent, fresh, sweet

Hyacinths are small plants whose spring-blooming flowers pack a robust fragrance wallop. Their short stature and intense fragrance make them good choices to plant along a fragrant pathway or at the front of a planting bed. Or plant them in containers, where they will be easy to see.

Plant hyacinth bulbs outdoors in the fall and they will bloom in early to midspring at the same time as many daffodils and early tulips. Because varieties are richly colored and available in almost every hue, including bicolor selections, hyacinths can be added to any cut flower garden and in any color palette. Hyacinths require a chilling period of two or four months in order to bloom. In warmer climates, it's a good idea to dig up and chill hyacinth bulbs over the winter before setting them out in the fall. Or treat them as annuals.

Hyacinths are also easy to grow and flower indoors by "forcing" the bulb. This means that you are tricking the bulb to bloom indoors instead of in the garden. To force a hyacinth bulb, place the bulb in a special forcing vase and add water. The bulb will wake from its dormancy and bloom inside your home in a matter of weeks instead of months in the garden. Be forewarned: the fragrance of a single bloom can permeate an entire room!

When choosing bulbs to plant, look for the largest bulbs. The bigger the bulb, the more stored energy the plant can access, resulting in larger, healthier spring flowers. Each bulb produces just one flowering stalk 8 to 10 inches tall, with a cluster of closely packed single and double star-shaped, small flowers. A heavy flowering stalk may need some extra support from a plant stake—or simply harvest the stalk for the vase. When plants are grown in clusters, the flowering stalks can support one another.

When harvesting a hyacinth, use caution, because some people are allergic to the hyacinth bulb and the slimy substance released when the stem is cut. If you are allergic or have sensitive skin, be sure to wear gloves when handling hyacinth bulbs and cut stems, and avoid touching your face until you have had a chance to wash your hands thoroughly. Harvest the stalk when half of the flowers are open at the base of the cluster. These flowers benefit from

mixed freesia

conditioning before being used in arrangements. Place cut stalks in a water-filled bucket in a cool, dark room for at least five hours before they are used. Hyacinth blooms typically last three to seven days in the vase.

Hyacinth is lovely in spring-inspired arrangements mixed with daffodils, *Ranunculus* spp., and other spring bulbs. When using them in natural scent projects, start with small amounts of the flower in enfleurage and tincture projects—a little can go a long way.

Iris spp., rhizomatous

Bearded iris	Landscapes, cut flower gardens
Zones 3–9 (selection dependent)	Floral, spicy, woody, chocolaty
Full sun	

With thousands of bearded iris cultivars available today, choosing only a few selections for your fragrant garden can be a challenge. Their pleasant fragrance can be extremely variable, with one cultivar, *I.* 'Gingersnap', even smelling like root beer! The colors of bearded irises can look as though they're straight out of a painting. There are so many wonderful colors to add to your garden, including pink, nude, mustard-yellow, rust, taupe, white, dark violet, burgundy, mahogany, and black. Several repeat-blooming selections flower twice a year. Bearded irises are collector's items for the cut flower garden.

Bearded irises need full sun and moderate watering regimens to thrive in the garden. Plant rhizomes shallowly in perennial garden beds and give this plant some time to shine. They are pretty low maintenance once established and become better and bigger as they age. Once they are done blooming, resist the urge to cut back the entire plant. They need their foliage to photosynthesize and store nutrients for growth in the following year. Their swordlike foliage provides great contrast to the flower heads in the cut flower garden and provides a nice visual aesthetic. Bearded irises attract primarily bees to the garden, though hummingbirds and butterflies will also visit the flowers. They also demand attention in the vase. Make room for their strong, straight stems and colorful blossoms. When flowers are spent in the vase, you can use the blooms in natural dye projects. Few flowers produce a woody fragrance, but bearded iris's spicy, woody fragrance is unique and adds a nice balance to floral blends when making tinctures and infusions.

'Immortality' bearded iris

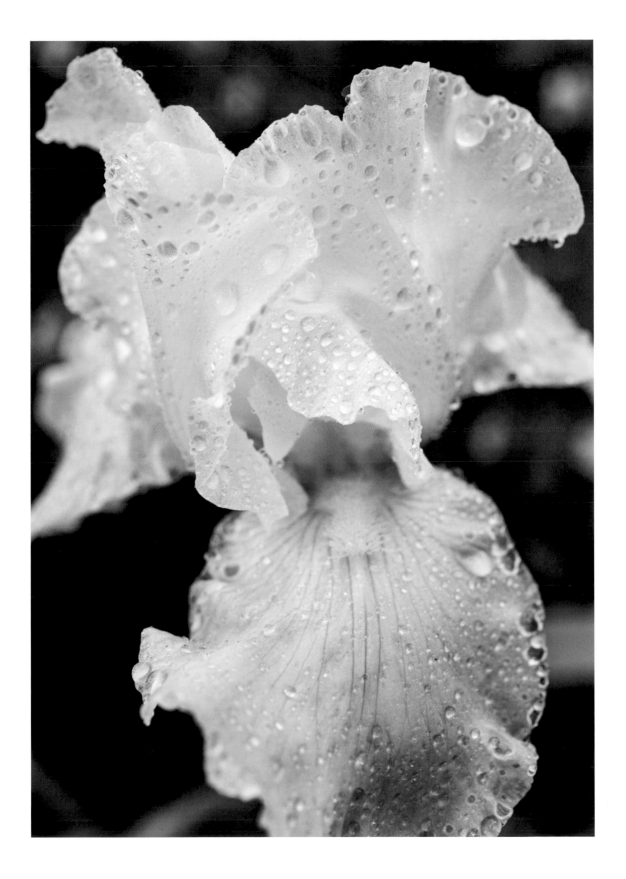

Lilium spp.

Lily
Zones 3–9
Full sun, part sun, part shade

Landscapes, cut flower gardens, containers

Honey, sweet, spicy, exotic

There is nothing subtle about a lily. Flamboyant, bodacious, and obscenely fragrant—we love this flower! When choosing a lily for the fragrant garden, start with your desired fragrance profile: do you want spicy or sweet? Then choose a color to fit your color palette.

Although lilies may look like tropical plants, they are hardy perennials that benefit from a winter chill to produce larger blooms. Several types of lilies all deserve space in the fragrant garden. Oriental lilies, with large, fragrant flowers that bloom in mid- to late summer, comprise the most fragrant selections. Orienpet lilies (also called giant lilies) bloom in early to midsummer and can be 6 to 10 inches across, and plants can be 3 to 6 feet tall. Trumpet lilies (including the classic Easter lilies) can be prolific bloomers in early summer. Other popular lilies include Asiatic lilies, but they have no fragrance.

Lilies are available in every color but blue. They may have spots or stripes, or they may be picotee (with dark edges). You could dedicate an entire garden to lilies and only scratch the surface of the possibilities. *Lilium* 'Star Gazer' is a lovely, pink, entry-level plant. If you want to take the next step in the lily realm, explore and search out a few favorites, including the double white–flowered *L.* Roselily Anouska, the dark pink–spotted 'Cat's Eye', and dark pink–striped Jaybird. Although the incredible number of lily varieties can be overwhelming, you really can't go wrong when choosing a lily for the fragrant garden, as long as it's fragrant.

In the garden, lilies prefer some shade around their roots, while the upper parts of the plants require sun. Flowers are typically six petaled, but shapes vary, including trumpet, funnel, cup, bell, bowl, or flat shapes. The flower heads are sometimes nodding, but most have reflexed petals in groups of three to more than fifteen on a single stiff, unbranched stem. Lilies are tall vertical growers that need only a little space at their base, but they need plenty of space to accommodate their large blooms. This means that lilies are well suited for placing in the back of the cut flower bed or in large container plantings. Taller plants may need staking when in full bloom because they can be top-heavy.

'Stargazer' lily enfluerage with coconut oil

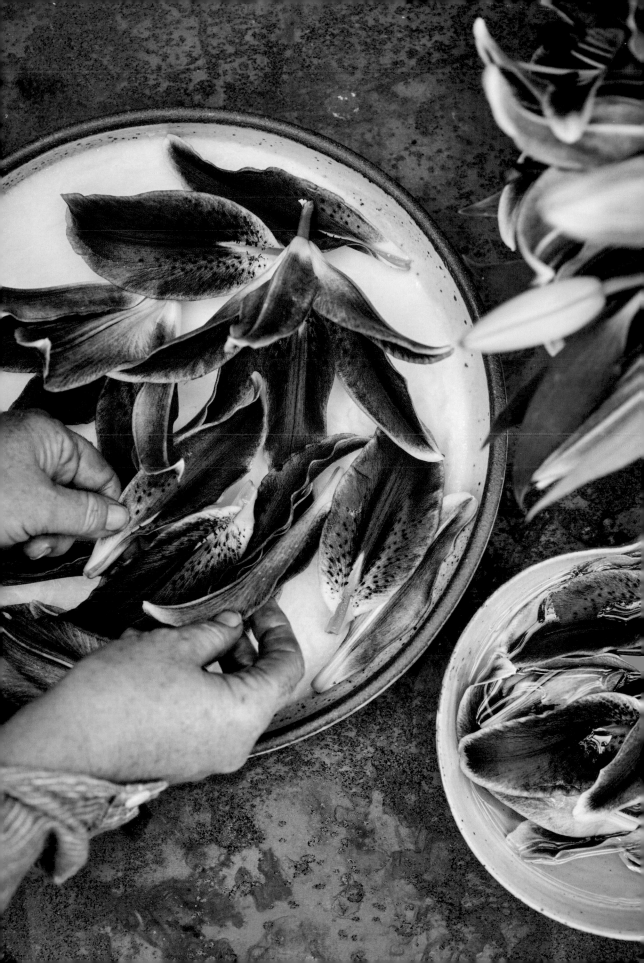

Most lilies grow from bulbs, but you can also grow them from seed. The best lily to grow from seed is the Formosa lily (*L. formosanum*), a classic, white, fragrant, trumpet-shaped lily. Unlike most lilies, Formosa lilies can be grown from seed and will flower in the first year. Most other lilies take two to six years to bloom when grown from seed, as opposed to bulbs, which flower in the first or second year. This is why planting bulbs is a good idea.

Harvest stems when the buds are just beginning to open and starting to show color. Lilies are good focal flowers with a long vase life in arrangements, and they can be very impactful even in a vase on their own. Be mindful of where you place arrangements that include lilies, as their fragrance can be overpowering. Even though some florists remove the lilies' pollen-containing anthers (which can stain clothing and skin), we keep them attached to experience all parts of the flower. We love it when the pollen ripens and stains the lily petals, creating a "full flower moment." For perfumery projects, you'll need to extract the scent from the large flowers. We suggest enfleurage in a shallow casserole dish that's large enough to keep the flowers intact.

Narcissus spp.

Paperwhites and daffodils	Landscapes, cut flower gardens
Paperwhites zones 8–10, daffodils zones 3–8	Sweet, jasmine, gardenia, hyacinth, spicy—or cat urine
Full sun	

Paperwhites (*N. papyraceus*) are the cilantro of the flower world. You either love their fragrance or hate it; there is no in between. For some, the flowers have a strong, gardenia-like scent, perhaps reminiscent of winter holidays; for others, they smell like cat urine. To determine whether you like their fragrance, buy a few varieties and force their blooms indoors. Once you get familiar with a bulb and determine its scent profile, you can either never buy paperwhites again or order more for the following year—and plant them freely in sunny spots throughout the garden.

The genus *Narcissus* includes not only paperwhites; it also includes spring-blooming daffodils, the bright, cheery faces that appear at the end of winter gloom to welcome spring. Daffodil flowers are not as pungent as paperwhites, but they are fragrant, including slightly sweet, very sweet, and even spicy scents.

Both daffodil and paperwhite bulbs can be forced indoors. Daffodil bulbs require a chilling period in order to bloom, but paperwhites do not. Both can be grown in containers, in planting beds, and throughout the landscape. Many will naturalize in the garden and are good choices for backyard garden beds, meadow plantings, and less manicured spaces in the garden. Like some humans, gophers are repelled by the scent of daffodils and paperwhites, so many organic gardeners traditionally line their fences or garden beds with these plants to deter these garden pests.

Stems of daffodils or paperwhites look great in a winter arrangement with pine and fir branches. Their fragrance mixes beautifully with rosemary and bay laurel in the vase and in a flower tincture.

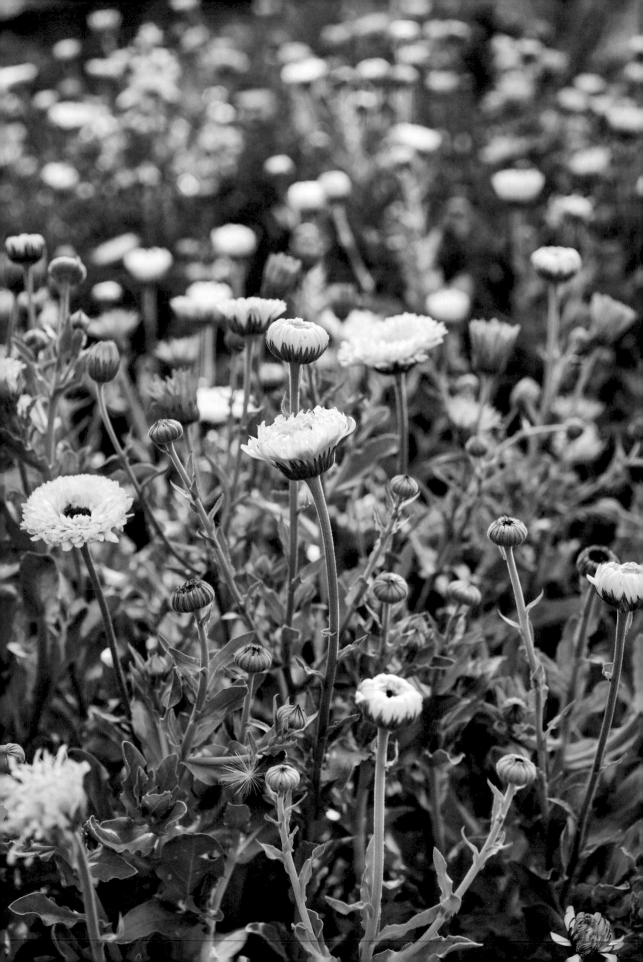

ANNUALS

Calendula officinalis

Pot marigold, calendula

Full sun to part shade

Landscapes, cut flower gardens, culinary and medicinal gardens, containers

Woody, musky, hay

Pot marigold is one of the easiest fragrant flowers to add to a garden, container, or planting bed, and its fragrance has a bite to it, which is interesting and unexpected from a plant that looks like a sweet, yellow daisy. It asks for a sensory double-take at first whiff. Easy to grow from seeds or seedlings, it blooms from spring through winter in warm climates and is not fussy about soil type or sun. As long as the soil is moist and well draining and the plant is not in deep shade, this garden staple will thrive.

Plants have an upright growth habit and are 18 to 24 inches tall, so they can be easily tucked among other fragrant flowers and plants. The open-faced flowers are similar to daisies and can be double and single, in a rich kaleidoscope of colors. Succession plant seeds from early spring through fall for continuous blooms.

Pot marigolds are prolific on several levels, including color variety, abundance of blooms, and medicinal value. A super-powered bloom, it is valued for its anti-inflammatory, antimicrobial, and immune-boosting qualities. You can use calendula-based infusions for scented lotions and balms and add its dried flowers in tub teas. We typically pair it with a more highly scented plant because the fragrance of calendula alone is not for everyone. Search out unusual selections such as peach-colored, double-flowered C. 'Bronze Beauty' and yellow-flowered 'Ivory Princess' for arrangements.

'Ivory princess', 'Bronze Beauty', and 'Indian Prince' calendula

Lathyrus odoratus

Sweet pea

Full sun to part shade

Cut flower gardens, containers

Citrus, orange, jasmine, sweet

With abundant, fragrant flowers in almost every hue, sweet peas are nostalgic, romantic, and endlessly useful plants for fragrant spring and early summer bouquets. Sweet peas should be near the top of any list of fragrant garden plants. If you're growing sweet peas from seed, you'll need to presoak the seeds for 24 hours in room-temperature water before planting. The seeds should swell up a bit; if one or two do not, continue to hydrate for another 24 hours. Once the seeds have swollen, they can be planted directly in the garden. Seeds can be planted in the fall for early blooms in many warmer climates or planted in early spring after the threat of frost has passed for summer flowers. The climbing vines need support from a trellis.

Sweet peas have a wonderful fragrance, but they are toxic and should never be eaten. This is important to note because each flower, after blooming, produces a pod similar to the pod of edible peas. For that reason, plant sweet peas separately from plants in your kitchen garden, and be sure to label the plant so that visitors do not mistake the sweet pea for its edible cousin.

Harvest flowers when half of the flowers on the stem are open, ideally in the morning before the plant is exposed to direct sunlight. Place the stems directly into a bucket or vase with cool water. Long-stemmed sweet peas are a key ingredient of spring arrangements, with beautiful tendrils and heavily scented flowers. Moody, dusky, and bright colors are great for arrangements. Look for tricolored, long-stemmed 'Enchanté'; the cream-colored, apricot-edged 'Mollie Rilstone'; or the lavender-inky 'Nimbus'. Their flowers can also be harvested for perfumery projects. Try making a sweet pea enfleurage or flower tincture.

'America'
sweet pea

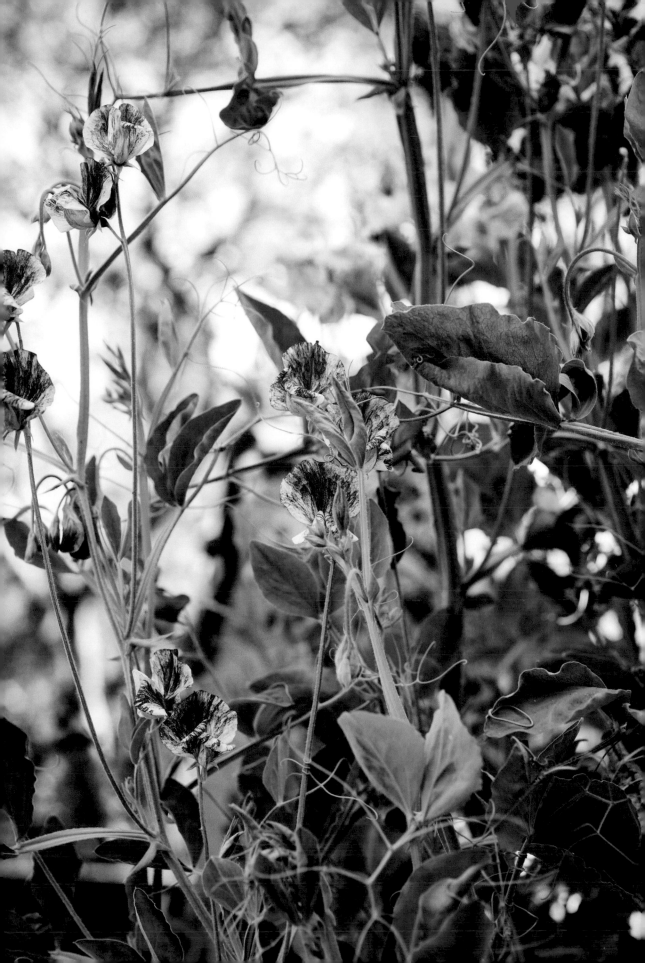

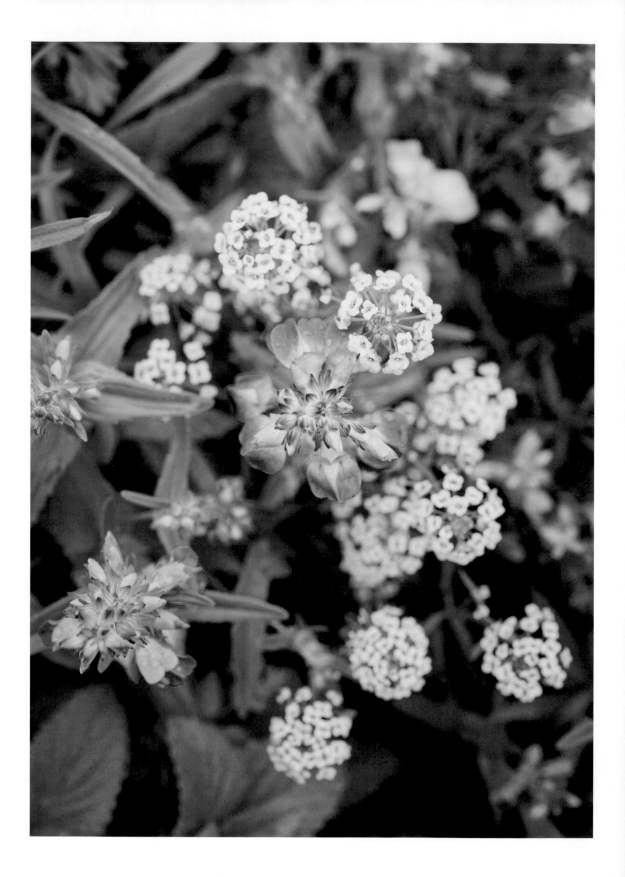

Lobularia maritima

Sweet alyssum

Full sun to part shade

Landscapes, culinary and medicinal gardens, containers

Honey

Sweet alyssum can be used as a ground cover, as an edger in a planting bed, or in a container, window box, or hanging basket. Plant it under citrus trees or other small trees in containers; it attracts pollinators, and its clump-forming habit does not crowd out the citrus. Sweet alyssum seeds are often included in pollinator-attracting wildflower mixes for meadow plantings. Although it is a short-lived perennial in zones 9 to 11, we treat this plant as an annual.

To include sweet alyssum in arrangements, you have to grow it yourself, because it is not typically sold for flower arranging. This little plant is a sweet addition to itsy-bitsy arrangements, nosegays, and boutonnieres. Add dried flowers to garden-grown potpourri, and use its flowers in oil infusions for balms and salves to add a bit of honey scent, along with citrus- and floral-scented plants.

Matricaria chamomilla

German chamomile

Full sun to part shade

Culinary and medicinal gardens, containers

Sweet, apple, herbaceous, earthy

The fragrance of German chamomile conveys a homey, cozy feeling, a sort of calming "sleep nectar." Its scent is unique and is at once recognizable. It has a gentle power to ease woes, soften nerves, and boost moods.

In the garden, this chamomile prefers the cooler weather of spring and fall. Because it doesn't thrive in the heat, scatter its seeds in your cut flower and herb beds where it will receive some shade in the summer. This annual happily reseeds, so leave a few flowers on the plant. German chamomile should always be included in cut flower and herb gardens. The perennial Roman chamomile (*Chamaemelum nobile*) is a shade-loving ground cover, with an equally beloved scent.

sweet alyssum and Chinese houses wildflower

Sprigs of German chamomile add bright white and yellow spots of color to summer arrangements. Use them for simple bouquets in a small vase placed

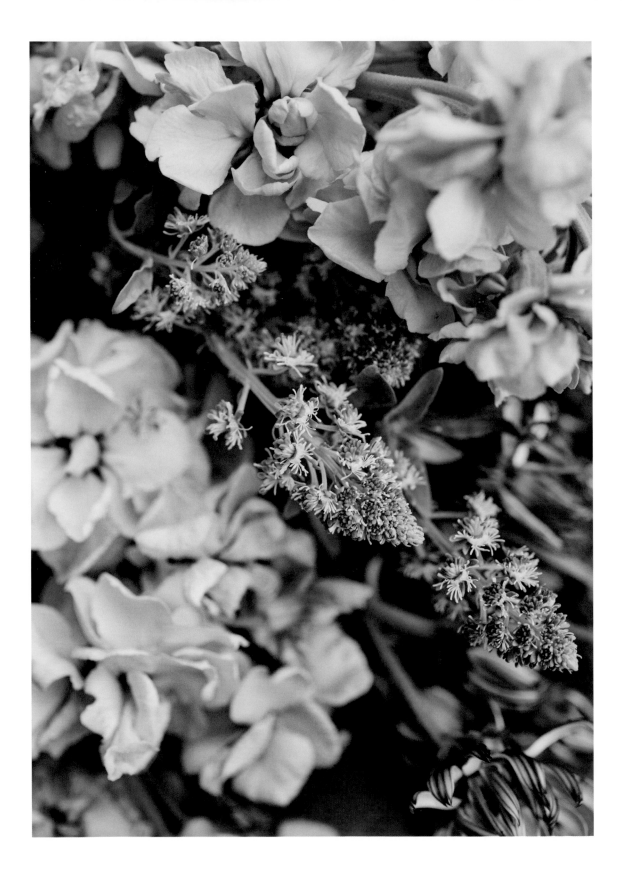

at your bedside, where you can appreciate their calming fragrance. German chamomile also holds its shape and color when dried, making it a wonderful addition to dried arrangement and wreaths. Its fragrance blends well with floral scents. Use it in oil infusions for hand salves and body balms. Add it to flower tinctures and—of course—it makes a fragrant, calming cup of tea.

Matthiola incana

Stock	Cut flower gardens, culinary and medicinal gardens, containers
Full sun in cool seasons, part shade in summer heat	Clove

Sometimes overlooked for the cut flower garden, stock is having a renaissance of sorts these days and is valued as both a cut flower and an edible flower. We love the sexy, bodacious, clove-scented blooms of stock, with single or double flowers that are tightly clustered on a single, straight stem.

Stock is a full-sun, cool-season annual that prefers spring and fall weather but will grow in summer, preferably in part shade. There is a stock for every color palette in the cut flower garden, including apricots, pinks, creams, pale yellow, antique brown, raspberry, and purple. If you plant stock from seed, the same seed packet may produce both single and double flowers. Be careful not to pinch back the plant or harvest early, thinking this will encourage more flowering, because after stock produces one flower spike, it is done. Harvest blooms when a third to half of flowers on the stem are open.

The double-flowered forms are often preferred by florists and are the best for the vase, while the single blooms are edible or can be used in perfumery projects. Stock's strong, straight stems make it easy to use in arrangements. The flowers can fill a vase and serve as both focal and secondary flowers with a long vase life. Stock flowers also hold their fragrance when dried. The easiest way to preserve the flowers is to hang stems upside down to dry in a cool, dark place. The deeper colored varieties maintain their color when dried and are beautiful for dried arrangements and wreaths. Dried stock flowers are also wonderful additions to tub teas and potpourri. The fresh flowers are easy to use in flower tinctures and oil-based infusions, adding their clovelike scent to your garden perfumery blends.

'Iron Apricot' stock and garden mignonette

Mirabilis jalapa

Four o'clock, marvel of Peru

Full sun to part sun

Cut flower gardens, containers

Lemony, fruity, honeysuckle, sweet, night-scented

In the late afternoon, these abundant, colorful, trumpet-shaped flowers exude a sweet, lemony floral scent in the garden. One of the plant's common names, four o'clock, describes its blooming time—from late afternoon through the night. When morning arrives, the flowers close.

Plant four o'clocks in cut flower beds or in other places where you can appreciate their sweetly scented evening blooms all summer long. Typically 2 to 3 feet tall, with a bushy growth habit, they are a good choice for the front or middle section of the planting bed. Plant them with flowering tobacco (*Nicotiana* spp.) along a fragrant pathway so you can enjoy a scented evening stroll through the garden.

While four o'clock flowers are open, hummingbirds and butterflies visit, but the blossoms are more often pollinated by nocturnal pollinators such as sphinx moths, which have long tongues to access the nectar inside the tubular flowers. Although the plants appreciate regular water, they are heat and drought tolerant, making them an excellent fragrant flower choice for gardens in drought-prone areas. The blooms wilt in the morning and then fade, becoming large, black-brown seeds. You can easily collect seeds for future sowings; otherwise, this plant will prolifically reseed and spread. If you garden in a colder climate, you can dig up the plants' black, carrotlike tubers to overwinter indoors before replanting them in the spring.

All parts of this plant are toxic if consumed. Flowers are traditionally used for a natural dye. Harvest blooms in the evening for casual arrangements on the summer dinner table. The pretty foliage with flowerless seed heads is particularly beautiful in arrangements and can be harvested in the morning.

Nicotiana spp.

Flowering tobacco

Full sun to part shade

Landscapes, cut flower gardens

Jasmine, night-scented

No night-fragrant garden is complete without flowering tobacco. These generous bloomers feature clusters of fragrant, star-shaped, tubular flowers in colors including white, rose, violet, mauve, and deep chocolate. This standout plant is carefree and easygoing, and it will bloom wherever you plant it in the garden. It is highly floriferous even in part shade.

Easily grown from seed, this plant comes in a variety of flower colors. We especially love *N. langsdorffii* cultivars 'Hot Chocolate' and 'Bronze Queen' for their dusky dark blooms, and sweet-scented *N. alata* 'Jasmine' is especially sensuous and fragrant. *Nicotiana mutabilis* is beloved for its white, pale pink, and rose-colored flowers that all bloom at once on a single stem.

Flowering tobacco's star-shaped flowers attract hummingbirds and butterflies in the daytime and hawk moths at night. If your garden experiences intense summer heat, plant flowering tobacco in areas with part shade. Many varieties can grow 3 to 4 feet tall, while others are more demure at 1 to 2 feet. Their height and sticky stems make most of them great choices for the middle to back areas of the cut flower bed. Flowers can appear a bit droopy during the day, but they perk up in the cooler hours of late afternoon, adding a warm sweetness to summer evenings or beneath an open window.

Its long stems are sturdy for arranging with a weeklong vase life, which makes up for their stickiness. Harvest stems when half of the flowers are open. Use the jasmine-scented blooms as secondary flowers in an arrangement, paired with roses. For perfumery projects, harvest flowers in the evening, when they are most fragrant.

Ocimum and O. basilicum cultivars

Flowering basils

Full sun to part shade

Cut flower gardens, culinary and medicinal gardens, containers

Tropical, sweet

With spikes of gorgeous, fragrant flowers that range in color from dark violet to white, flowering basils are a showy and productive addition to the fragrant cut flower and edible garden. Unlike the annual Genovese basils, the flowering basils are sterile and bred for their flowers, and they will continue to grow—rather than stopping growth, going to seed, and dying—while flowering. Flowering basils can be grown as a perennial in zone 10 and as an annual everywhere else. They are a bit more cold tolerant than most basils and will usually last in the garden until the first frost. Because they are sterile and do not produce seed, they must be propagated from cuttings.

Ocimum basilicum 'Magic Mountain' and *O. basilicum* 'African Blue' grow to 3 feet tall and need full to part sun. Mix them in generously throughout the back of the cut flower planting bed, giving the plants space to grow large. Plant in several groups of three or five throughout a long planting bed, or add them at the ends of beds to create a dramatic entrance planting. *Ocimum basilicum* 'Wild Magic' usually tops off around 18 to 24 inches, making it a great option to plant along a fragrant pathway or at the edge of a raised bed.

We line pathways and planting beds and fill containers with flowering basils so that we can activate their fragrance as we walk through the garden. To say that flowering basils attract pollinators is an understatement. The bees get drunk on its nectar and do not care when we run our hands through the blooms beside them.

It's no surprise that the fragrant blooms of flowering basil can be used for excellent garden arrangements. The key to creating a long-lasting arrangement is to harvest basil during cool mornings and keep the cut plants out of direct sunlight. Do not harvest in the midday heat and sun or when the plant is dry, because the cut stems will wilt immediately and often will not rehydrate. Flowering basil's beautiful purple-tinged stems make a lovely greenery base in arrangements, where they create a beautiful rhythm. Flowering basil makes a great filler and is also beautiful on its own in a single-specimen arrangement. If the cut stems do not wilt, they will last one or two weeks in a vase and often

'Mountain Magic' flowering basil harvest

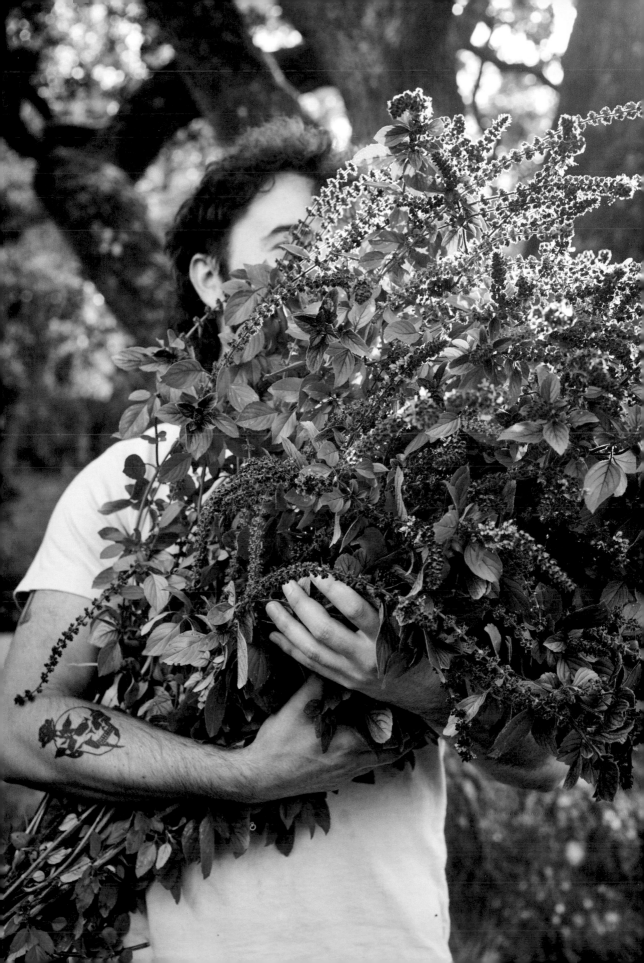

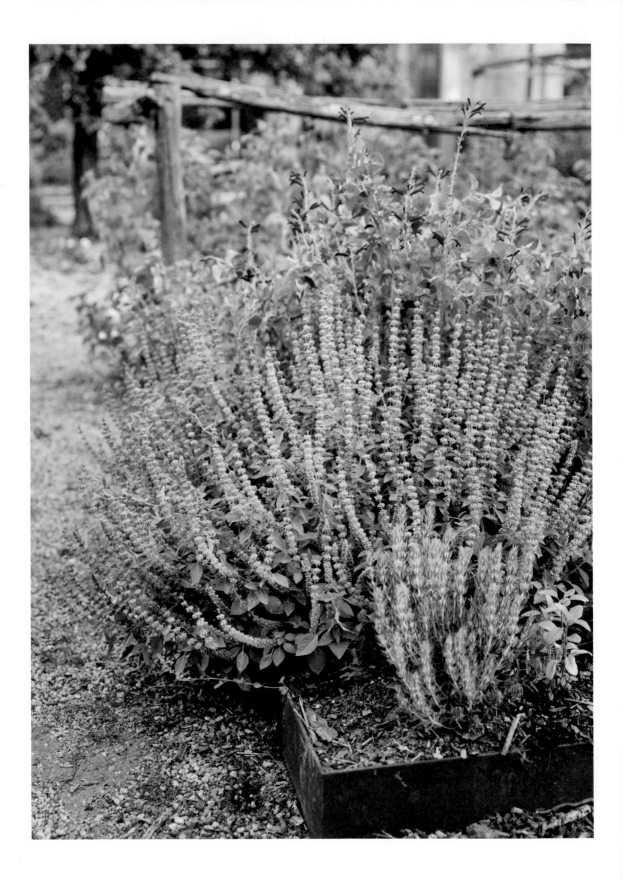

start to grow roots. You can plunk the rooted stems into a pot to start a new basil plant. Their tropical scent pairs well with citrus, floral, and woody scents. It's a fantastic plant for flower tinctures, enfleurage, and oil infusions.

Ocimum tenuiflorum

Holy basil, tulsi
Full sun to part shade

Culinary and medicinal gardens, containers
Balsamic, cinnamon, peppermint, clove, basil

Holy basil thrives in full sun with low to moderate water. In most areas, this heat-loving herb should not be planted prior to June, when temperatures are most favorable. It needs ample heat for leaf growth. Favorite variations of this species include Krishna tulsi (dark green to purple-green leaves), Rama tulsi (green leaves), and Vishnu tulsi (purple-green leaves), which are all named after Hindu gods and used in Ayurvedic medicine. We plant them all in the summer garden, though we prefer Rama tulsi for its forgiving versatility.

For the most potently fragrant leaves, begin harvesting them in midsummer and continue harvesting throughout the summer and fall. When the plant starts to bloom, holy basil makes a good filler plant for fragrant arrangements. Pair it with other favorite scented herbs, including calendula, blooming oregano, German chamomile, and lemon verbena, in a striking medicinal arrangement. Enjoy them in a vase for a few days to a week, and then remove the plants, cut off the stems that are no longer fresh or that show water decay, tie them together with twine or string, and hang them to dry in a cool, dark place. In a couple of weeks, when the leaves and flowers are dry to the touch and crumbly, combine the dried materials in a bowl for a fragrant garden tea blend, or use them to make an oil infusion for hand salve. Doubly good.

tulsi basil and
'Tangerine' sage

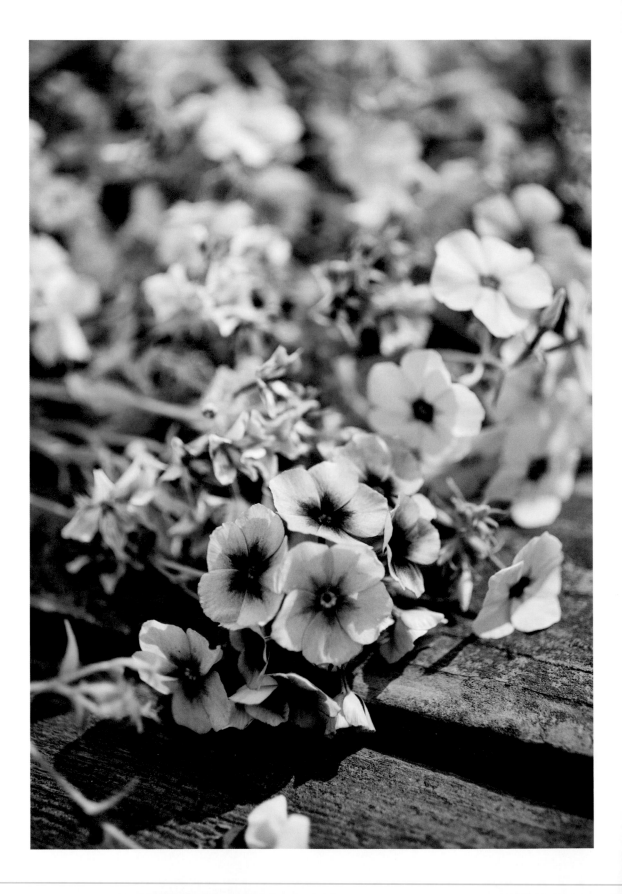

Phlox drummondii

Phlox	Cut flower gardens, containers
Full sun	Lightly sweet

With star-shaped flowers and a subtle, sweet fragrance, *P. drummondii* is an old-fashioned classic in the cut flower garden. Billowy in nature, phlox can be planted in drifts in areas with full sun. Plants grow 12 to 18 inches tall and almost 12 inches wide, with abundant flowers atop green foliage.

You can start seeds early in a greenhouse or sow seeds directly in beds in the early spring. Phlox will bloom gloriously all summer and into fall, dying once frost arrives. The colors are incredible! Flowers in butterscotch, caramel, and cherry-pink cover the 'Cherry Caramel' cultivar. The blues and whites of 'Sugar Stars' remind us of faded blue jeans, and the buff-colored 'Crème Brûlée' is a must for the dusky cut flower palette. They are all stunning.

Harvest stems with fully open flowers. Phlox works well in arrangements, adding a lightly sweet fragrance. Although you can pinch and deadhead phlox to increase blooms, we prefer to use the wispy, leggy stems in arrangements, which add a romantic touch and allows for a longer stem in the vase. Phlox mixes well with the floral scents of robust flowers such as peonies and roses.

Reseda spp.

Mignonette	Cut flower gardens, containers
Full sun to part shade	Musky, spicy, sweet, ambrosia

A truly delightful fragrant flower for the cut garden or container, this plant's common name, mignonette, is from the French word *mignon*, meaning "dainty"—like a dainty steak. Small spikes of white, pinkish, or dusky brown-red flowers are wisps of fragrance when they bloom.

Mignonette mixes well with all color palettes in the cut flower garden, especially the dusky palette. It is not a showy flower, but a diminutive spike of flowers that packs an ambrosial floral punch. This is a great plant for the front or middle level of the bed or in a container, where you can appreciate its small flowers. Depending upon the variety, flower spikes can grow tall, especially white

'Cherry Carmel' phlox and 'Sugar Stars' phlox

mignonette (*R. alba*). It is easy to grow and does best when directly seeded in the garden. Mignonette reseeds easily and you can collect its seeds for future sowings. Look for garden mignonette (*R. odorata*) for its dusky colored flowers.

Harvest mignonette when flowers are half open on the spike. The flowers last a week or longer in the vase. Spent flowers are also beautiful in bouquets, and the dried seed pods are as interesting as the blooms. Mignonette mixes well with other plants in arrangements as a secondary flower, gestural touch, or filler; or harvest for a single variety arrangement. Flower scents are extracted via infusions.

Tagetes spp.

Marigold	Cut flower gardens, containers
Full sun to part shade	Musky, earthy

Marigolds are covered in fragrant blooms from late spring to fall. Their earthy scented foliage can be pungent, and some find it bitter, but don't let this discourage you from planting this garden staple! It is a fantastic plant for attracting beneficial insects and repelling unwanted mosquitos in the garden.

Marigolds can be grown in any garden in full sun. Easygoing, heat tolerant, deer resistant, and in constant flower until first frost—it's easy to understand why marigolds are favorite garden annuals. Direct sow seed in the spring after the last chance of frost. Plants typically germinate quickly (four to seven days), but watch out for snails and slugs that will devour seedlings in the spring. Deadhead spent blooms to keep the plant blooming throughout summer and fall.

Marigolds are best known for the varieties with large, double-flowered, pleated blooms. Among these, look for *T. erecta* Coco, *T.* 'Day of the Dead Golden Yellow', and 'Zenith' series French marigolds. Colors include white, butterscotch, yellow, orange, and burgundy red. The heirloom types have graceful, wavy stems and open, single blooms. Search out *T.* 'Villandry' and *T. erecta* cultivars 'Burning Embers' and 'Harlequin' for cut flower gardens. Plant them in the middle to the back of the bed; many grow to 3 feet tall.

Harvest flowers for garlands and arrangements in summer and fall. Marigolds can also be used in natural dye projects and have medicinal antiseptic and skin-healing properties, making them a good choice to include in fragrant hand balms and salves, which we appreciate as gardeners and florists. Their bitter, earthy scent is perfect for our medicinal scented projects.

'Villandry' marigold

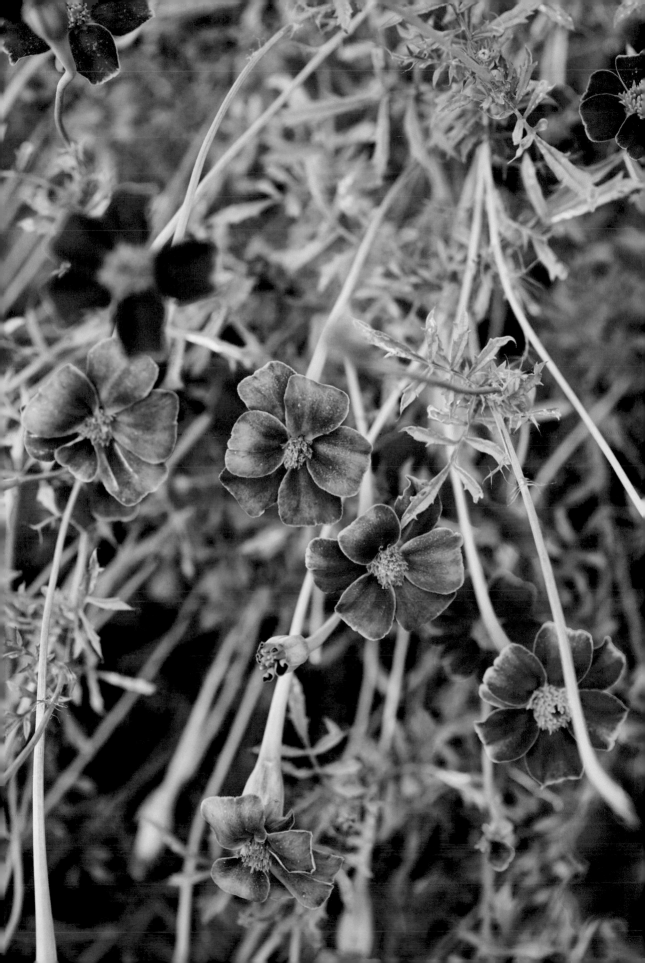

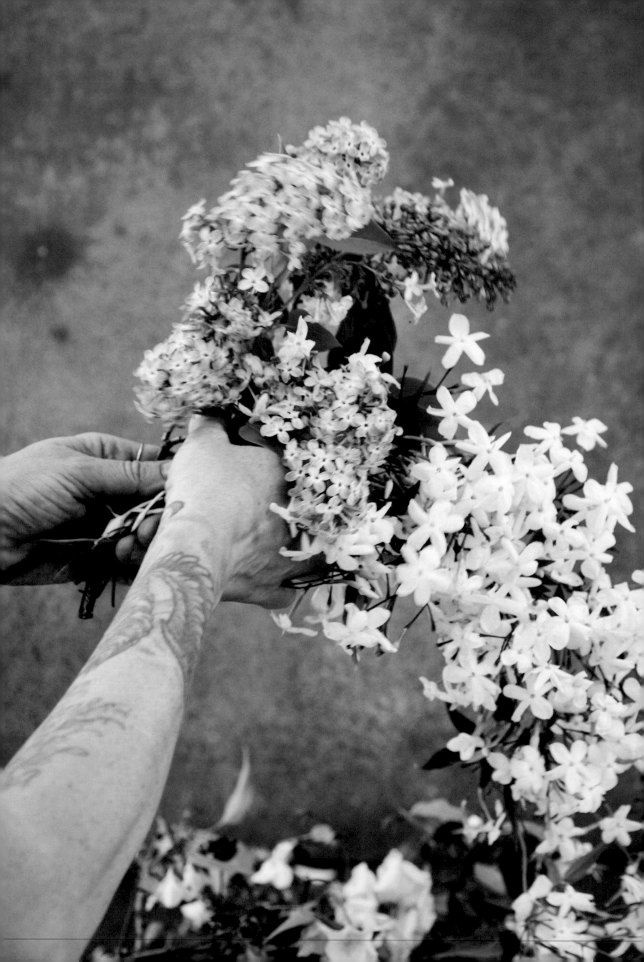

CHAPTER THREE

HARVESTING & ARRANGING FRAGRANT FLOWERS

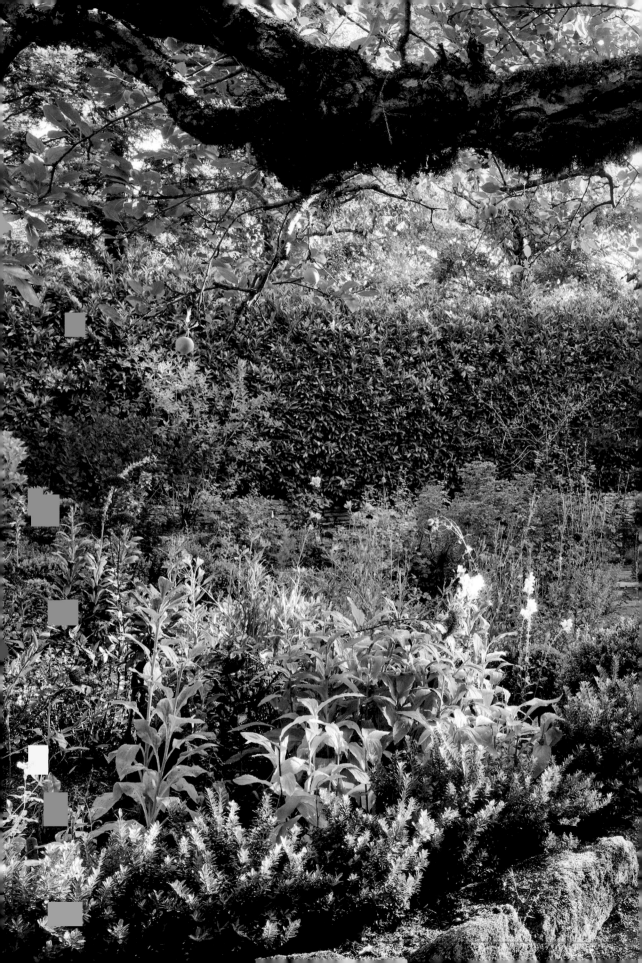

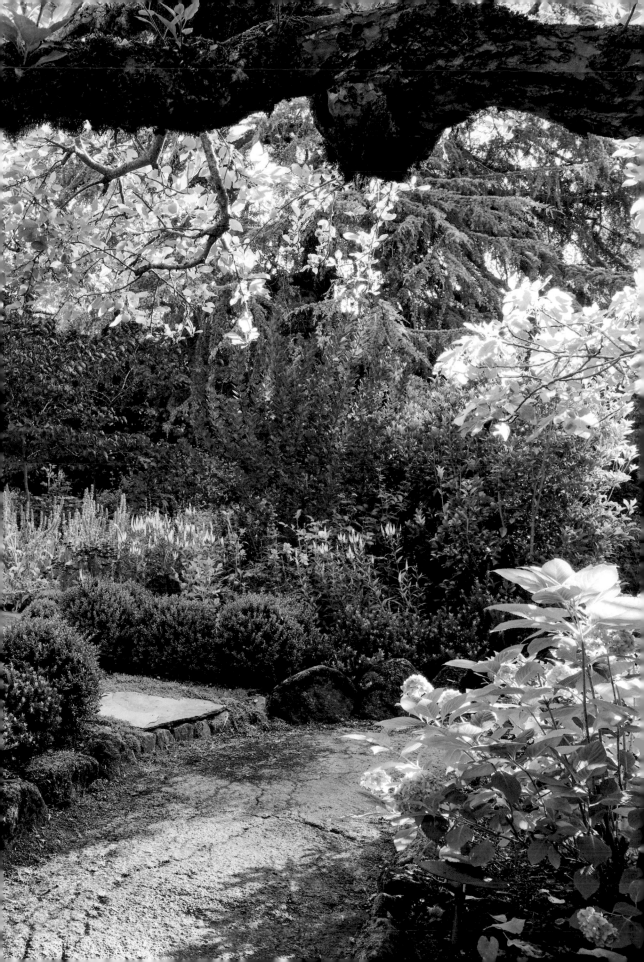

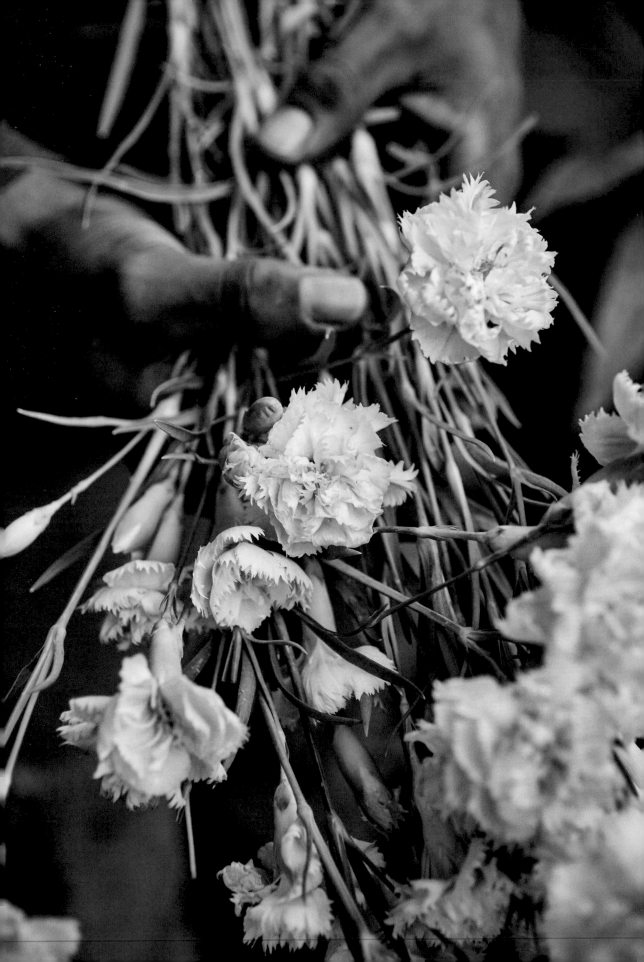

Fragrant cut flower beds (see page 23) provide endless sources of inspiration for floral arrangements. Bring along hand pruners as you visit these beds or wander through the garden, and you'll likely find yourself harvesting and arranging the flowers in your hand as you go. If you've made three cut flower beds organized by the flower types used in arrangements—dedicating at least one bed each to focal flowers, secondary flowers, and filler—it becomes even easier to harvest and arrange using the grouping technique (see page 24). Keep the focal, secondary, and filler materials together in their respective groups to begin the arranging process while you're still in the garden. After you've visited the dedicated annual beds, look for flowers and foliage to harvest in the greater landscape and perennial beds, adding bits of fragrant plants to the arrangement in your hand. Then you can transfer the arrangement from hand to vase.

In addition to identifying the flowers and foliage that will serve as focal flowers, secondary flowers, and filler in the arrangement, you also need to consider their scents. Take inspiration from perfumery as you combine fragrant plants for the vase. Most combined scents consist of three notes in the following order:

Top note: floral or citrus

Middle or heart note: spicy or musk

Base note: woody or earthy

The top note is the first fragrance you encounter in a perfume or an arrangement. It sets the tone of the overall combined fragrance and should transition well into the middle note. The middle note adds complexity and provides a longer lasting fragrance. The base note holds the entire scent combination together and is usually the last fragrance to evaporate.

Keep these three notes in mind as you harvest for the vase. A fragrant arrangement will have a more pleasing aroma and appearance if the plant scents and colors are complementary and combine well together, instead of clashing, with too many highly scented plants and colors. Note that if you

'Chabaud La France' carnation

don't like the fragrance of a plant in the garden, you will probably not like it indoors in a vase either. A plant's fragrance is intensified inside, where it is not competing with other garden scents. Sometimes a neutral-scented flower (one with no scent) is helpful to add to a fragrant arrangement when you are including multiple intensely scented blooms; it can provide space between fragrant flowers so that each can have its moment to shine.

HARVESTING & CONDITIONING

Harvest stems in the early morning before the heat of the day sets in or at dusk after temperatures have cooled. Keep them properly hydrated after being cut to prevent the blooms from going limp.

Fill a bucket three-quarters full with cool water and bring it with you into the garden. After you've finished harvesting and arranging the flowers in your hand, place the stems directly into the bucket. It's okay if the leaves or blooms are submerged because this will help with the rehydration process. If you wait too long to put the flowers in water, the stems will form a seal on their cut ends, making it more difficult for the stems to absorb water. If you have spent a long time meandering through the garden harvesting flowers and greenery, you can recut the stem tips before placing them in water to help with hydration.

In a perfect world, your bucket of freshly cut stems, including all the ingredients (focal, secondary, and filler) for your arrangement, will be placed in a cool, dark room for at least five hours before they are handled again. This gives the stems time to rehydrate and will lengthen their life in the vase. If you can cut flowers a day before you arrange them, waiting twelve hours between harvesting and arranging is ideal.

Woody stems of plants such as lilac and mock orange have a difficult time absorbing water after they are cut. Making a diagonal cut on the end of the stem helps the woody branch absorb more water. Or you can smash the last inch or so of the cut ends with a mallet to break them up, which also helps with absorption.

Cutting Tools

A good pair of heavy-duty pruners or shears is essential, along with a pair of smaller floral snips for skinny, delicate, or hollow stems. Loppers or pole pruners are good to have in your tool supply for cutting thicker woody stems or branches.

BUCKET AND VASE CARE

Clean buckets and vases are important for cut flower arrangements. Leftover particles of dirt and rotten plant material can enter freshly cut stems and clog the xylem tissues—the thin, strawlike tubes that draw water up into the stem. If the xylem becomes clogged, the bloom will prematurely go limp and will never properly hydrate.

Arrangement Care

Place your finished arrangements out of direct sunlight in a cool room, away from a heating source. Nothing ruins an arrangement faster than direct sunlight and heat. Every day, tip the old water out of the vase into the sink and add fresh water to the arrangement. If your sink has a sprayer attachment, use it to flush out the vase before adding fresh water.

Arranging Tips

Alethea likes to harvest groups of stems (focal, secondary, filler) from the garden and place them in the water bucket at the same time to retain the groupings or bunches. Then, after she adds the flower bunches and groups into a vase, she adds a few single stems to add dimension and movement to the composition. This simple grouping technique can make a big impact with any size of arrangement and helps you create a natural, fresh-looking arrangement.

Before you begin arranging, know where you'll be placing the arrangement inside your house. If it will be placed on a mantel, the arrangement can be one-sided, with the flowers featured in the front of the arrangement. If the arrangement is for a coffee table, where it will be visible from all sides, the flowers should be arranged to look good from every angle.

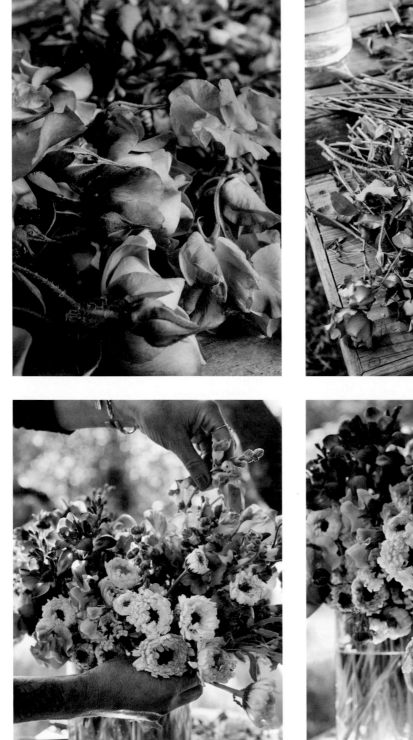
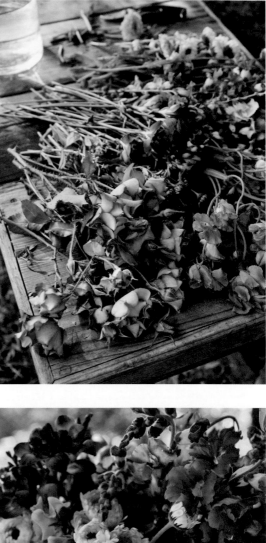
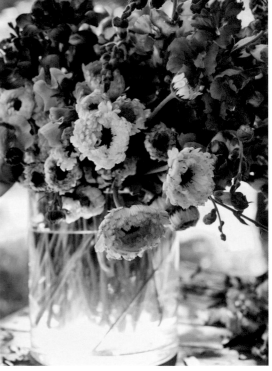

Here are a few more of Alethea's favorite tips to keep in mind when creating your own garden-grown arrangements:

- Place heavily scented arrangements in entry ways or room entrances to welcome folks into your fragrant home.
- Include herbal or lighter floral scents in arrangements for the kitchen and dining room table to avoid the fragrance clashing or competing with food aromas.
- Although eco-friendly floral foam (used to hold flowers upright in the vase) is available, most traditional foam is composed of toxic, carcinogenic ingredients. Because prolonged exposure to this material can lead to health problems, we never use it. Instead, we prefer to use floral tape, pin frogs, or wire cages, all of which are available at craft stores. Or we use a greenery base method to hold flowers in place.
- It's okay to add packaged flower food to vase water; it's simply plant food and an antibacterial substance that will prolong the life of the flowers. We stick to using clean, cold water in our arrangements and make sure to add fresh water to the vase daily, as cut flowers tend to drink quite a bit. You may have heard some suggestions about adding substances to the water to prolong flower life, such as adding a penny or lemon lime soda. Although we don't subscribe to any of these methods, for some, they have a very personal meaning. If your grandma told you to add a penny to the vase, it doesn't hurt to do so!
- Before adding flowers and greenery, fill the vase about halfway with water so it doesn't accidentally overflow while you work.
- Remove foliage from the lower parts of plant stems that will sit below the vase's water line. Keeping this extra plant material out of the water will help the arrangement stay fresher longer.
- As a rule, the stems should be about one-and-a-half times the height of the vase. So, for example, if the vase is 12 inches tall, the flower stems shouldn't be taller than about 18 inches.
- If you're using a pin frog or another method to hold flowers upright, and the flowers fall to the sides of the vase as you're adding the first stems or bunches, either the stems are too long or the opening of the vase is too large.
- Make sure that when you add flowers into the vase, the stems reach the bottom of the vase or very close to it. If the stems are too short, they may not be in water and will die or go limp quickly, shortening the arrangement's life.
- You'll know when the arrangement is done because you'll either be out of flowers or you won't be able to add any more flowers to the vase (or, Alethea's favorite, you're happy with it as it is).
- Once you've finished the arrangement, add more clean, cold water to the vase, filling it almost to the brim.
- Most importantly, have fun.

FRAGRANT GARDEN ARRANGEMENTS

Use these step-by-step arrangement directions to help you create beautiful and balanced scented arrangements. Keep in mind that you don't need to use every single ingredient mentioned in a recipe. Instead, we hope these arrangements will help inspire your own ideas, so that you can get out in your own fragrant garden and start arranging! You can swap out what grows in your garden for some of the flowers used here. By arranging garden-grown flowers, you can avoid wasting beautiful cut flowers: rather than having to purchase a big bunch of flowers just to get a single, special flower you want for an arrangement, you can simply go outside and harvest what you need.

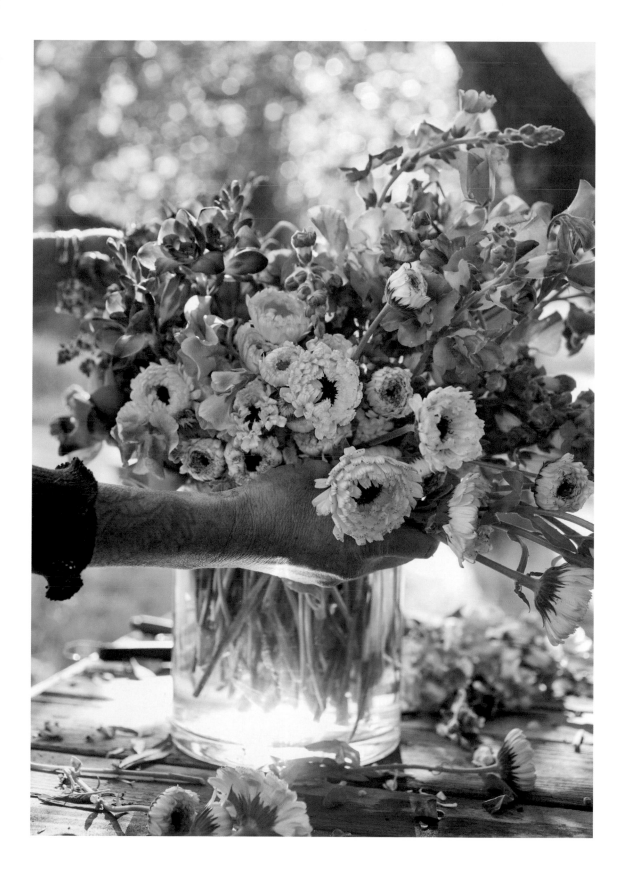

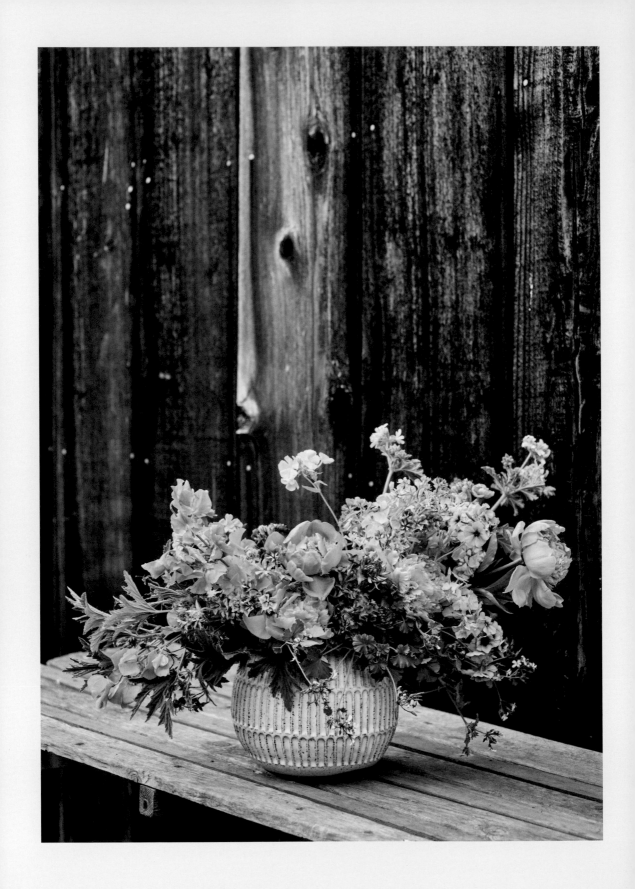

SPRING EXPLOSION

7 long stems 'Mabel Grey' scented geranium

7 long stems 'Nutmeg' scented geranium

3–5 stems peonies

15 stems 'Crème Brûlée', 'Cherry Caramel', and 'Sugar Stars' phlox

20 stems 'Bronzed Beauty' calendula

3–5 stems 'Vintage Brown' and 'Iron Apricot' stock

15 stems 'Big Blue' sweet peas

Spring often seems to arrive suddenly, with a magnificent explosion of flowers and scents in the garden! This arrangement captures and celebrates spring. Garden-grown arrangements preserve a moment in time, when all the plants used in the arrangement emerged in your garden together. This romantic arrangement by Alethea can be easily assembled with the help of a few lush, pleasantly fragrant peonies (see page 64 for recommendations) and the delicate, yet heady, aroma of sweet peas. You really can't go wrong with this combination of spring ingredients. Peonies are the focal flowers. Secondary flowers include sweet peas and stock, which add a spicy fragrance that complements the floral peonies. Phlox and calendula are more lightly scented secondary blooms that add complexity, and the scented geranium foliage completes the arrangement in the role of filler. This composition would be perfect as a table centerpiece or as an entryway showpiece in your home.

CONTINUED

Choose a bowl-shaped vase with a wide opening for this composition so that all of the juicy blooms can spill out over the sides of the vase.

Create a base with the scented geraniums, the designated filler plants. Add all the stems of the two geranium cultivars to the vase in bunches. Bundle two or three stems of each type of geranium, alternating between the types as you work your way around the opening of the vase. Make sure that the lowest leaves on the stems rest on or over the edges of the vase and that no leaves are below the water line. Cross the stems in the vase, creating a nest for the flowers to be placed in and supported by the filler plants.

Place your focal flowers, the peonies. We often harvest peonies when they are in bud and not quite open, as this prolongs their vase life. After the peonies open, their large, ruffled blooms will take up more space. Don't crowd the peonies as you place them in the vase, and be sure to leave plenty of room in the arrangement for the flowers to open. Cut the stems of one or two peonies to be slightly taller than the rim of the vase, and place them in the front of the arrangement so that they can provide a beautiful focal point to showcase the biggest blooms. Add the remaining, longer stems of peonies on the left and right sides to add dimension and depth.

Fill in empty spaces in your arrangement with bunches of secondary flowers, including phlox, calendula, and stock. Vary the lengths of the stems so that some bunches will be taller than others. This will break up the height cluster of flowers for a more natural feel. Leave one or two stems longer to add some height and balance to the overflowing scented geraniums.

Because of the delicate nature of the sweet pea blooms, wait to add them until you are almost done with the arrangement. Place the sweet pea stem bunches to one side of the peonies in the front, making sure to leave their stems longer so their delicate flowers aren't damaged.

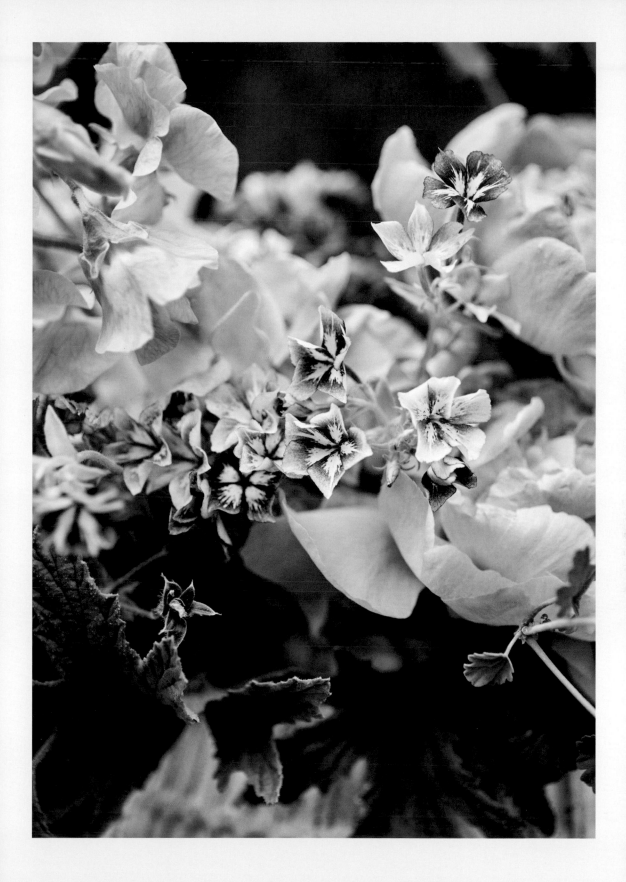

LAFAYETTE SUMMER

4 long stems 'Gleam Salmon' nasturtium with flowers and foliage

5 stems 'Wild Magic' flowering basil

2 stems Purple Bumble Bee cherry tomato

2 long stems flowering tobacco

5 stems 'Villandry' and 'Day of the Dead Golden Yellow' marigolds

3–4 stems unscented 'Apricotta' cosmos (*Cosmos bipinnatus* 'Apricotta')

If spring arrives in an explosion, summer takes its time heating up the garden. The summer garden is abundant with highly fragrant flowers that can be used in arrangements along with cuttings from the edible garden. In this arrangement, the tropical floral fragrance of flowering basil pairs nicely with the herbaceous and pungent fragrance of cherry tomato stems with their fruit and flowers intact. Open-faced 'Villandry' marigolds add a spicy note along with their more traditional marigold cousin, 'Day of the Dead Golden Yellow'. A peppery nasturtium is used as the arrangement's filler. We love how nasturtiums trail over the edges of our garden beds, and we used that as inspiration for this arrangement, with long stems of nasturtiums that flow out and over the vase. Flowering tobacco adds a sweet floral note, and the arrangement is finished off with some unscented cosmos to fill in the spaces between all of the heady summer scented blossoms.

Harvest these plants while they are long and leggy, just as they are in the midsummer garden. Alethea uses long stems to make tall arrangements that are reminiscent of a garden meadow, where all of the plants grow wild but come together to make a beautiful composition. If one of the flowers has gone to seed on a stem of multiple blooms, you can leave the seed heads. Include all parts of the plant—even these seed heads—in this garden-inspired piece.

CONTINUED

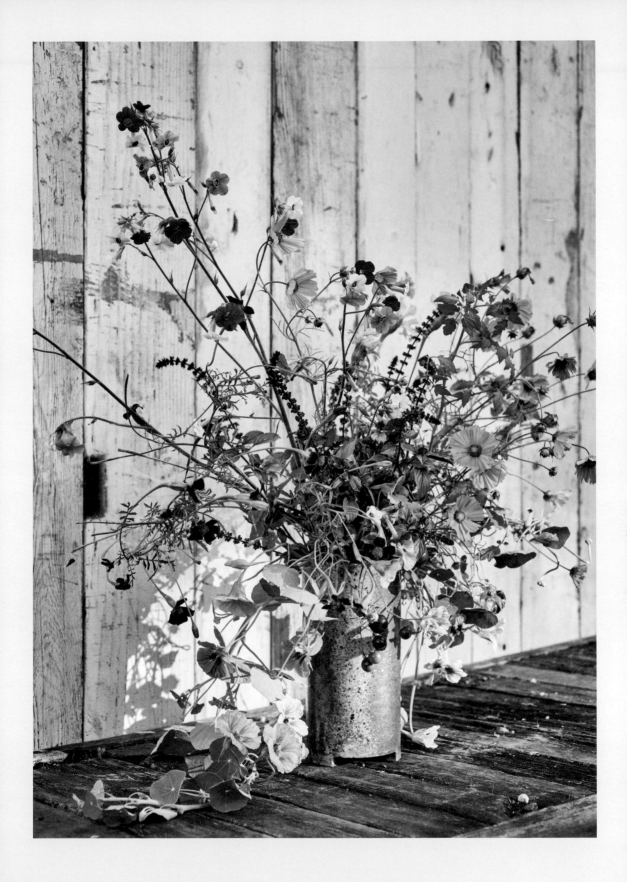

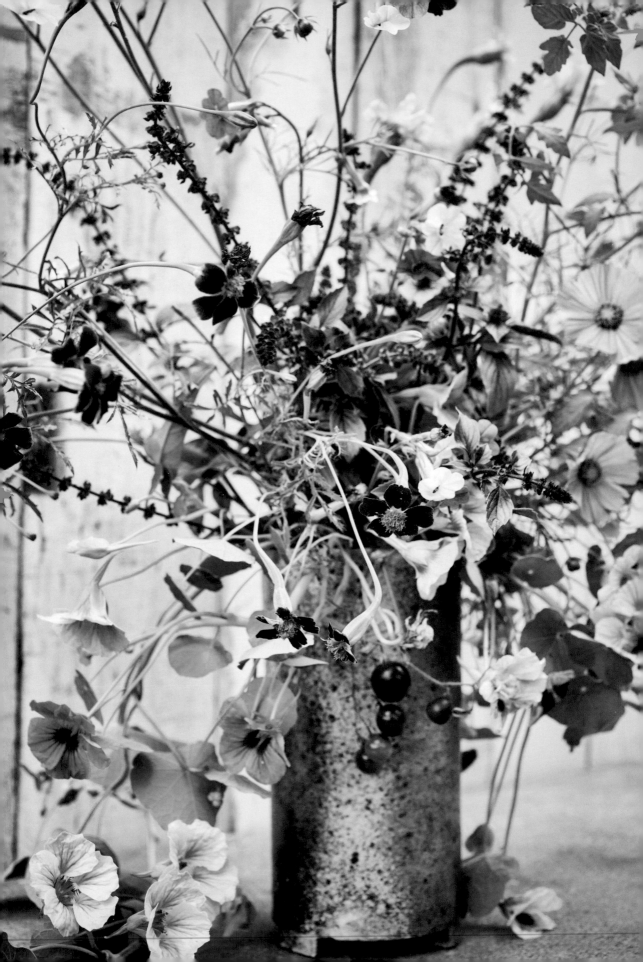

Choose a tall vase that can accommodate the long stems, with an opening of 5 inches or less wide. These summer blooms all have skinny stems, so a smaller vase opening will help keep the arrangement upright.

Place groups of nasturtiums as filler on either side of the vase, making sure to remove any foliage that will fall below the water line inside the vase. Cross the stems to create a nest of stems that will support the focal and secondary flowers.

Add the taller filler stems of flowering basil. The fragrant purple foliage with conical shaped flowers helps to create a taller base for the thin-stemmed flowers to follow.

Gently place the taller focal stems of cherry tomato and flowering tobacco. Place these stems at slight angles, rather than straight up and down.

Fill out the arrangement with groupings of the secondary marigolds in similar bunches—separating any strong, competing scents with groupings of the unscented cosmos. Don't overthink this type of arrangement—it is meant to be wild.

A ROSE CELEBRATION

8–10 stems honeysuckle

22 stems mixed garden roses, including flower buds or rose hips, plus open flowers

10 stems blooming Clary sage

5 small bunches blackberry sprigs, 2–5 sprigs per bunch

10 stems late-season oregano with dried seed heads

We invited our friend and fellow florist, Juliette Surnamer, to Stefani's garden in late summer to explore fragrant flowers with us. Many of Stef's roses were in full bloom and inspired this arrangement. Harvest half-open blooms in the morning—that's when garden roses are ready for pollination and therefore at their fragrance peak. Half-open blooms also have the added benefit of a longer vase life. We also celebrate the rose's abundance by including sprigs of unopened rose buds as a secondary flower in our arrangements. While not yet fragrant, these sprigs have a beautiful and unique texture and can add movement to the arrangement. By growing your own roses, you can include all parts of the flower's life stages in your arrangement, which is a beautiful way to celebrate the garden's most famous fragrant flower.

When rose petals drop, the seed-filled pod (the rose hip) is exposed. If left on the stem, rose hips will grow and develop lovely orange or red colors as they ripen. During the summer, as roses grow quickly, we prune and remove dead flowers (deadhead) from the roses in the garden to promote more flower growth. But sometimes we miss a spent flower here or there, and we harvest the rose hips that have begun to develop to use in arrangements. At the end of autumn, we typically stop deadheading our roses as winter nears and encourage the rose hips as a late-season treat for bouquets and as an ingredient for tea.

Clary sage (*Salvia sclarea*) is a wonderful accompaniment to roses, as its fragrance has a warm, sweet, herbaceous scent. It pairs well with all of the scented roses but especially well with musky and fruity scented varieties. We included sprigs of blackberry that grow near Stefani's climbing roses on a garden fence. The not-quite-ripe fruit adds a beautiful visual component to the arrangement, playing the role of an unscented ingredient to separate the stronger scents. When using berries in arrangements, harvest unripe sprigs— ripe berries can drop and create a bit of a mess as the arrangement ages.

CONTINUED

Honeysuckle and long, leggy stems of oregano serve as fillers in this arrangement. Honeysuckle's beautiful, bright green foliage and sweetly scented flowers are welcome in all of our summer arrangements. Most herbs like a good pruning in the summer, and oregano is no exception. After it goes to seed, its stems make great additions to any arrangement with a spicy scent and beautiful color. If you have the patience, avoid pruning your oregano too early in the summer. Not only will beautiful seed heads develop, but the foliage of the spent flower heads will fade to a tawny, golden color as the plant focuses its energy into growing new foliage at the base.

Although we don't typically wear garden gloves while arranging flowers, when we're working with this many roses, we wear them. We also remove any large thorns on the roses that may create trouble while arranging. You will need access to all sides of this arrangement as you create it, so make sure that you can walk around all sides of your work table.

For this arrangement, choose an urn-style, footed vase with a wide opening to accommodate a large arrangement. Prepare the vessel by creating a flower frog from coated chicken wire to hold up and support the roses' heavy flower stems.

Here's how to make a flower frog from coated chicken wire.

Cut a square piece of wire about 3 to 4 inches wider than the vase's opening.

Bend the wire into a ball, shaping it to fit in the vase's opening, and place it inside the vase. Make sure that the top of the wire ball doesn't show above the rim of the vase. Stretch floral tape across the top of the vase to attach the flower frog to the vase; this will help keep the frog from moving as you add large, heavy stems. Even though you will be covering up the tape with long stems of foliage and flowers, you should use only as much tape as necessary. Avoid placing long pieces of tape on the vase that won't be covered with plant material.

Create small bunches of honeysuckle and place them in the vase as the base filler. Set aside two to four especially beautiful stems with flowers to add later. Place the honeysuckle bunches in three or four separate locations along the edges of the vase, leaving space between the groupings for secondary flowers. Make sure the stems are in the flower frog. Place the longest stems at slight angles at the front of the arrangement and on one or both sides.

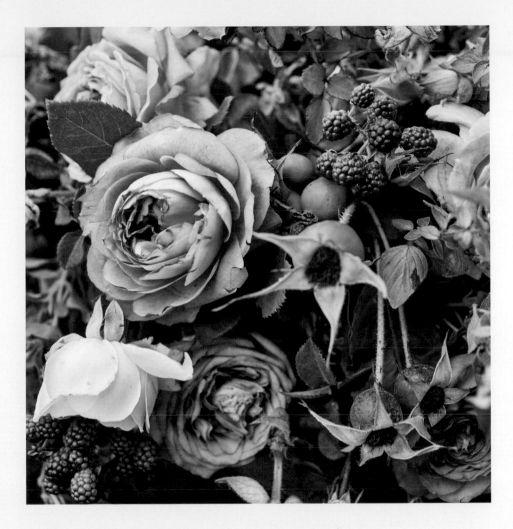

Create multiple small bunches of roses, each composed of three flowers in different colors (in our case, each bunch included flowers in pink, orange, and creamy white). Add flower bunches throughout the arrangement for a fresh-from-the-garden feel. If you've harvested an especially beautiful bloom, place it front and center in the vase. Place longer stemmed roses at the sides.

Group together three stems of clary sage and place them among the rose groupings, breaking up the groups. Place longer stemmed clary sage bunches so that they fall over the edges of the vase. Intersperse more clary sage throughout the arrangement, and add a bunch of sage to the back of the arrangement, angling the stems toward one side or the other (not directly in the center).

Continue to fill in the spaces between the rose groupings with shorter stemmed blackberry sprigs, placing them near the flower heads to fill in spaces. Fill any remaining spaces with the oregano and any leftover honeysuckle filler—again repeating placement with groupings for better visual impact.

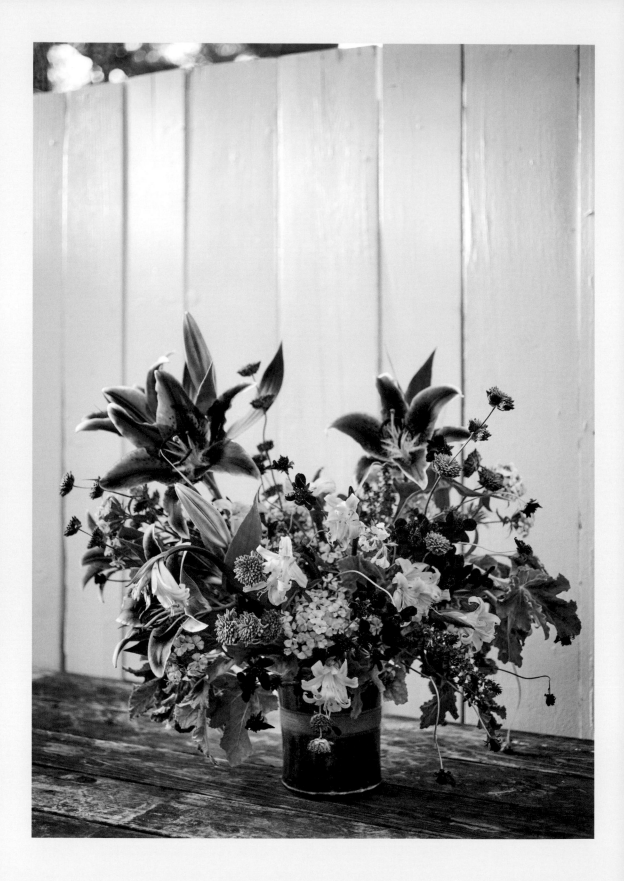

LILIES & CHOCOLATE COSMOS

5 stems peppermint geranium

3–4 stems oriental hybrid lily (such as 'Stargazer' or 'Jewel Star', which is pictured in our arrangement)

15–18 stems chocolate cosmos

10 stems sweet William

7 stems belladonna lilies

3–5 stems flowering basil

9 stems Cleveland sage dried seed pods

Maybe it's because we were teenagers in the 1980s, but we have always loved the color combination of pink and brown. There are many aromatic pink flowers in the fragrant cut flower garden—most of our favorite scented blooms have pink varieties that are easy to find and cultivate. But brown? There is really just one brown (actually dark maroon) flower—*Cosmos atrosanguineus*, Chocolate cosmos. Its petals are not only brown, but they smell like chocolate, and they pair both aromatically and visually with the sweet scent of pink lilies and sweet William. Juliette explored Stef's garden, cosmos in hand, to find the perfect companions for this chocolate-inspired arrangement. The focal flowers are, of course, the lilies. Few flowers command as much attention in a vase. For the secondary flowers, we turned to belladonna lilies (sometimes called naked ladies), with intensely sweet blooms. These are actually not a lily at all, but an amaryllis (*Amaryllis belladonna*)! A South African native, these pink-flowered beauties are beloved for their fragrance and their easy growing habit. We also included sweet William blooms to repeat color and fragrance throughout the arrangement.

And, of course, the chocolate cosmos! When arranging with chocolate cosmos, we find that adding fewer groups with a lot of stems creates a greater visual impact (the delicate flowers can get lost otherwise) in an arrangement. You can also add a few chocolate cosmos as gestural bits to the arrangement—placing long stems in one direction, with the flower heads far from the center of the arrangement.

Brown seed pods of highly fragrant Cleveland sage repeat the brown theme in the arrangement, adding a nice contrast to the large lilies. If the dried pods have retained their scent, it will be much fainter than fresh stems of sage and will not compete aromatically with the lilies. Lastly, for filler, we

CONTINUED

use a few sprigs of flowering basil. When harvesting the basil, we chose stems with long flower heads that showed off their dark stems, complimenting the dark hues of the cosmos and seed pods. We also used peppermint geranium (*Pelargonium tomentosum* 'Chocolate') as filler. Many of the flowers in this arrangement have long stems without foliage, so the large, ruffled leaves of scented geranium are needed to cover and soften the space between the vase's edge and the flowers. The geranium's minty aroma pairs well with the fragrance of chocolate cosmos and the lilies, and its ruffled brown, variegated leaves are perfect visual cues that bring the arrangement all together!

Choose a crock-style, ceramic vessel. Make a chicken wire flower frog for this arrangement to support the lilies' large flowers and heavy stems. Cut a piece of coated chicken wire that's roughly the size of the vessel's opening, and shape it into a ball. Place the chicken wire ball inside the vessel, making sure that it rests at the bottom of the vase.

The geranium leaves are large and are quite impactful when placed in the vase on their own, so there's no need to use bunches of stems in the vase. Place the longest stem of geraniums on one side, overhanging the vase. Place two other stems in the vase, one toward the center and the other opposite that stem. Set aside the two remaining geranium stems to add later, if needed.

Next, place the focal lilies. Vary the height of two stems so that one is shorter than the other. Place these two stems on one side of the vase. On the other side of the vase, add a third stem that's slightly shorter than the tallest lily stem.

Make a large bunch of chocolate cosmos (with about 70 percent of the cosmos stems) and place the bunch in front of the single lily on one side. Tuck in sprigs of sweet William and stems of the belladonna lilies in between and surrounding the larger lilies. Break up the pinks by adding smaller groupings of the chocolate cosmos. Leave a few stems long and place them so that they "float" out of the arrangement.

Add the flowering basil stems between the belladonna lilies and chocolate cosmos, and then add the dried seed pods of Cleveland sage near the larger lily heads, facing the same direction the flowers are facing. Add the last two stems of scented geranium to the arrangement if needed to fill spaces or to cover an edge of the vase.

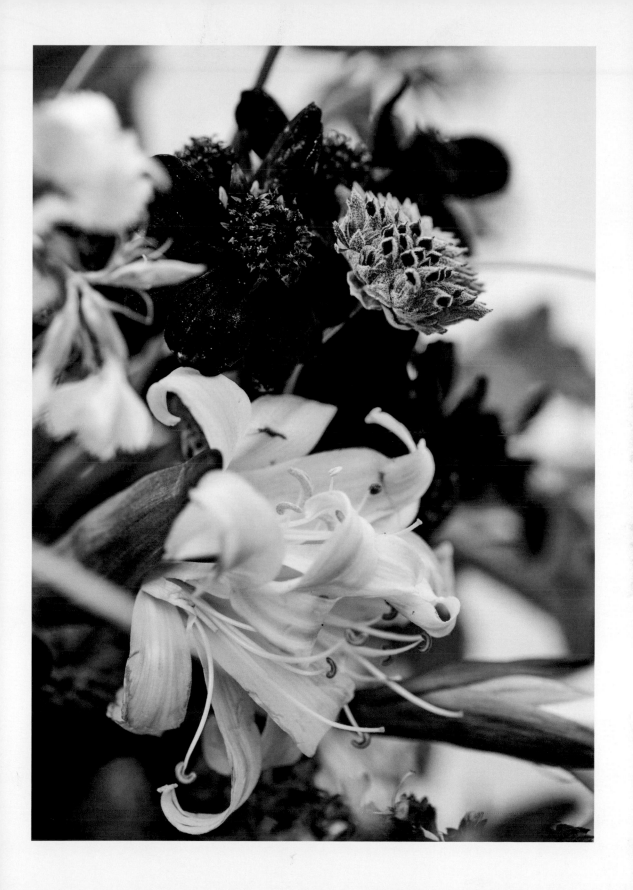

WORKING HERB WREATH

3–4 bay laurel branches,
18–24 inches each

4–5 bay laurel stems,
about 12 inches each

10–12 long stems oregano,
with flowers or seeds

12–15 stems lavender

10–12 stems German chamomile

4–5 stems feverfew

4 stems bee balm

4 stems scented geranium

We include many herbs and edible flowers in our gardens and flower arrangements for a reason: they are some of the most fragrant plants in the garden! When summer is at its peak, our gardens are overflowing with these plants. This project is a wonderful way to create a decorative and purposeful arrangement in the form of a wreath. Alethea refers to it as a "working wreath" that serves as a spice cabinet of sorts: we snip off bits of the wreath during the year to use in cooking. It's an enjoyable way to display and store the preserved herbs and edible flowers you have grown throughout the year.

You'll need wall space in your kitchen or pantry for hanging the wreath. When you have these herbs at your fingertips (especially during the winter months when the garden is not so bountiful), your cooking and tea-making will evolve and grow—just like your garden! You'll need medium-gauge florist's wire and natural kitchen or garden twine for this project. And make sure you have plenty of space to create this wreath—a large kitchen counter, indoor tabletop, or a shady outdoor table should give you the room you need.

Bend the longer branches of bay laurel into a circle and bind the ends together using florist's wire. You can also use your favorite natural gardening twine, but the wire is better at keeping the wreath frame in place as the branches dry.

With the remaining edible herbs and flowers, make small bunches in your hand, with each including four or five stems of the same herb or flower. Tie the bunches together with wire or twine and set them aside, keeping the like varieties together. You'll end up with multiple bunches of oregano, lavender, and chamomile.

Using twine, secure the bunches onto the bay laurel frame. We like to group several small bunches of the same herb or flower together, making our way around the form, transitioning from one to the next. If you have lots of one particular herb, you can repeat a grouping with different herbs and flowers between two similar herb groupings. Continue in this fashion until you have covered the frame.

CONTINUED

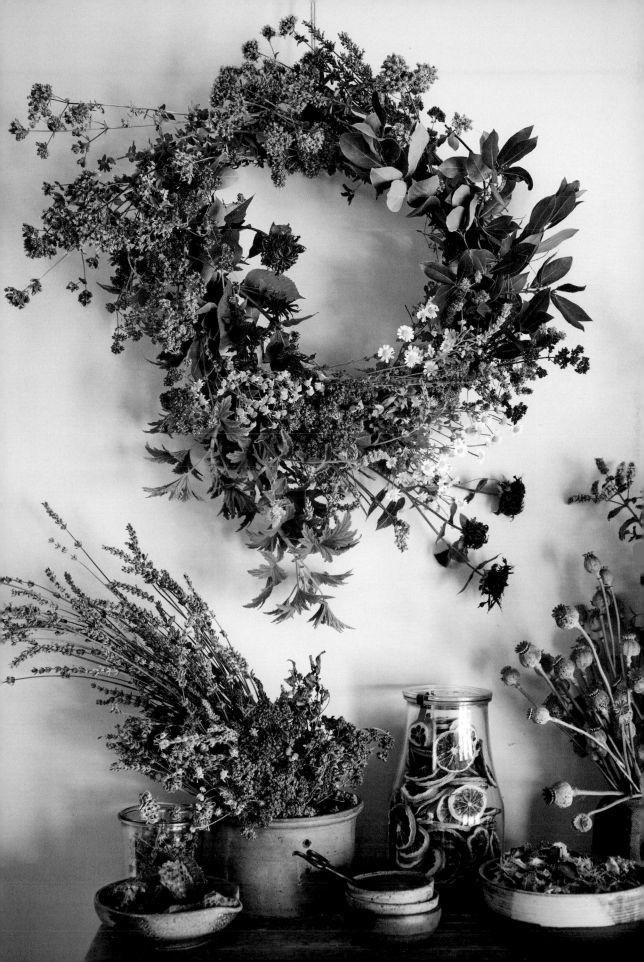

Cut a longer piece of twine to attach to the wreath and hang it for drying. Tie the ends of twine together to create a loop. Then lay the wreath on top of the twine so that one end of the twine loop is visible in the center of the wreath and the other end is outside the wreath. Take the looped end in the center of the wreath, bring it up over the wreath frame, and thread it through the loop of twine outside the wreath. Pull to tighten, and you are then ready to hang the wreath.

Choose a location with good air circulation, away from direct sunlight. The herbs will typically dry in about two weeks. When they are dry to the touch and crumble easily, the drying process is complete. If an herb or flower is still pliable and bends easily when touched, continue to let the wreath dry.

Keep a pair of scissors nearby to harvest the dried herbs directly from the wreath as needed for cooking and making tea. Or harvest all of the herb bundles when dried, moving the dried herbs into mason jars for storage. Then start the process again with fresh new herbs and flowers! The bay laurel wreath frame can be used over and over again, so there's no need to take it apart.

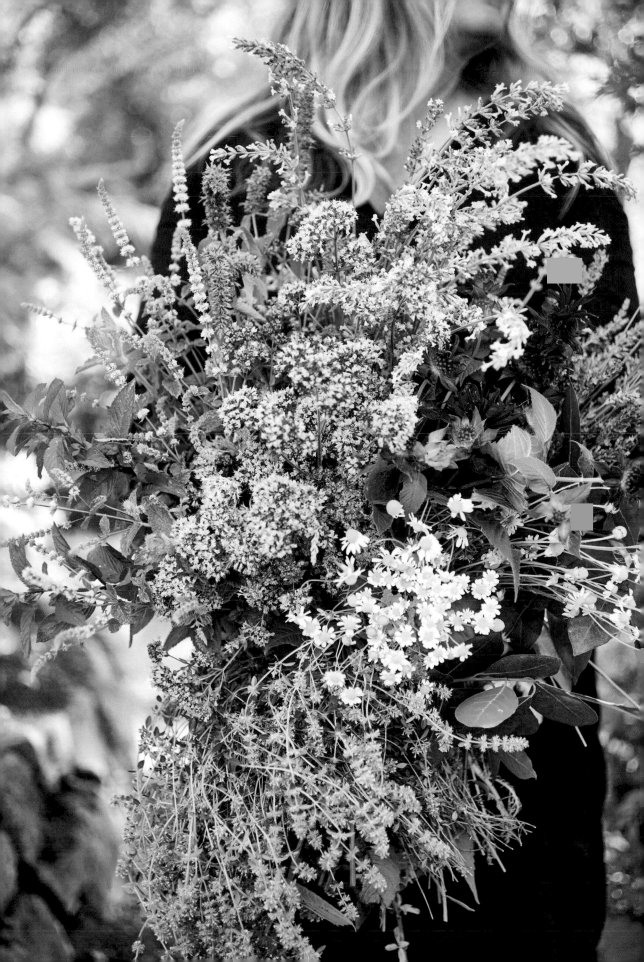

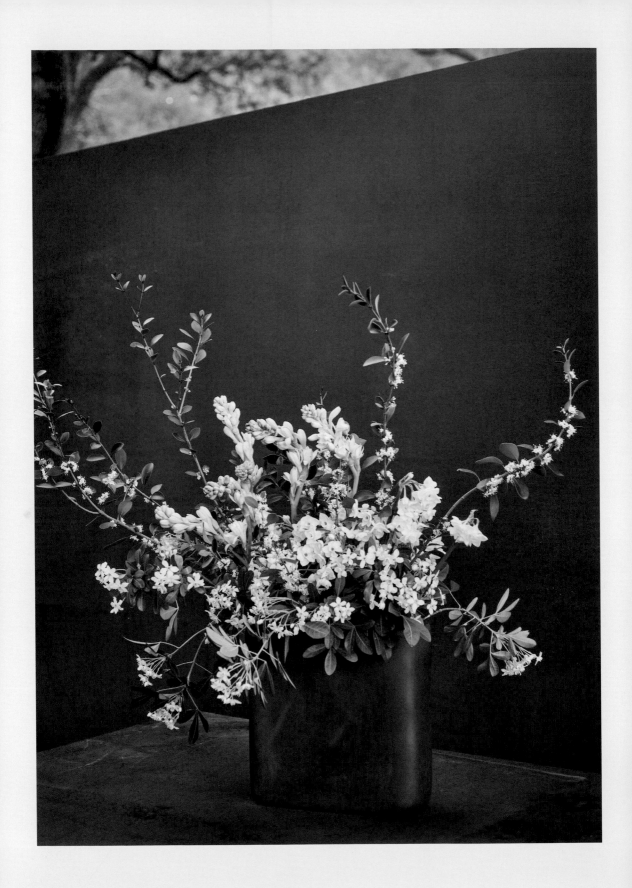

WINTER WHITES

5 wide, multistemmed branches
of Mexican orange

5 stems tuberose

12 stems paperwhites, with flower
buds less than halfway open

7–8 single, slightly curving branches
of sweet osmanthus, 1–2 feet each,
with at least half the flowers in bud

As the garden transitions to winter dormancy, we appreciate the more diminutive but no less aromatic flowers of our winter-blooming shrubs and bulbs. These fragrant plants are rarely found in florist's shops, so if you plant them in your garden, you will have abundant winter blooms. This arrangement, like the garden this time of year, is all about the greenery and white blooms. We harvest armloads of sweet osmanthus and stems of Mexican orange, filling our vases and using the winter fragrance for garlands and wreaths. Place a simple sprig of osmanthus in a bud vase by your bedside and it will perfume the bedroom, with a fragrance that surpasses that of any holiday candle.

This arrangement includes fragrant paperwhites, which are easy to grow indoors in a simple container. In areas with warmer climates (zones 8 to 11), paperwhite bulbs will thrive and naturalize when planted directly in the landscape. There are many fragrant paperwhites to explore, and not all of their flowers are white. For this arrangement, however, Alethea kept to the classic white palette, embracing all that is subtle and beautiful about these white blooms. Sprigs of tuberose round out this winter celebration. We grow this bulb in our greenhouse just for this sort of occasion.

CONTINUED

Use a tall vase with a narrow opening for this branch-heavy arrangement. Add the three widest branches of Mexican orange as the base filler. The branches should fill the bottom half of the arrangement and extend over the edges of the vase. Cross the branches inside the vase, creating a nest for other branches and stems.

Add the focal tuberoses, placing varying lengths in the center of the arrangement and to one side of the vase. This will leave space on the opposite side of the vase for the paperwhite stems. Place the tuberose stems diagonally so that the flower heads point toward one side of the arrangement.

Fill the empty side and a bit of the center space with paperwhites, making sure that the flower heads are above the Mexican orange and below the tuberose flowers.

Fill out the arrangement with the osmanthus branches, placing the longest branches on either side rather than at the center.

Add the two remaining Mexican orange stems to the arrangement to fill holes and pointing to the sides of the arrangement or toward the tabletop. Fill out any last remaining spots with the remaining stems of paperwhites. Vary their lengths so that a few stems are well above the Mexican orange blooms.

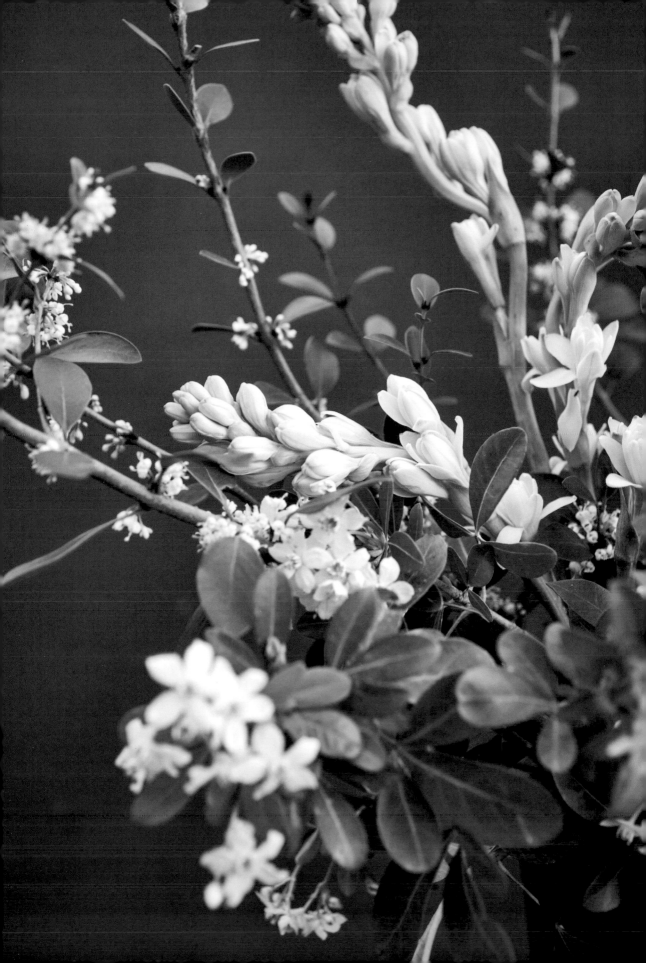

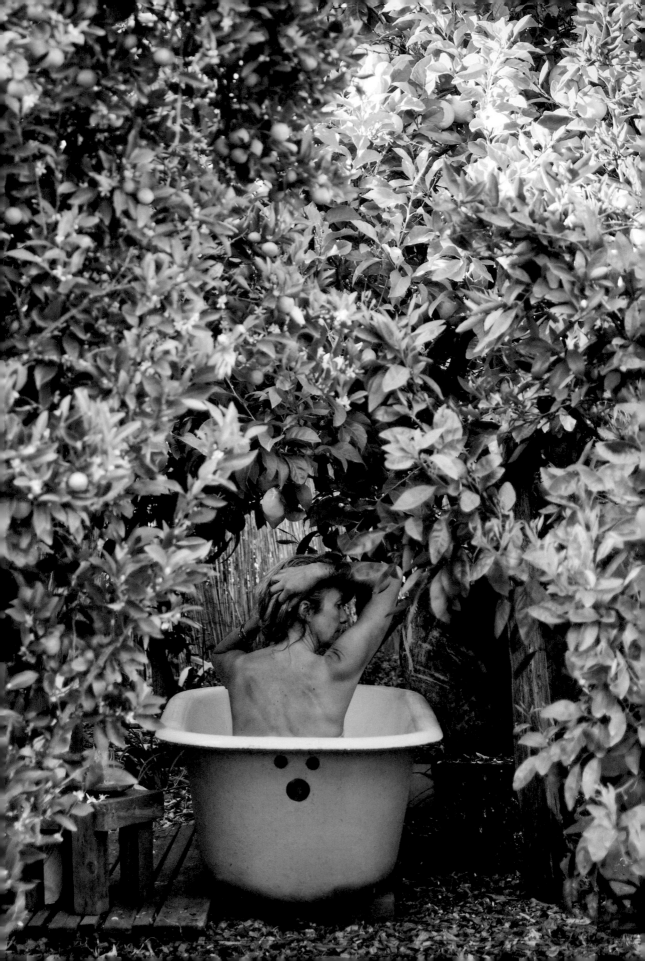

CHAPTER FOUR

CAPTURING & PRESERVING FRAGRANCE

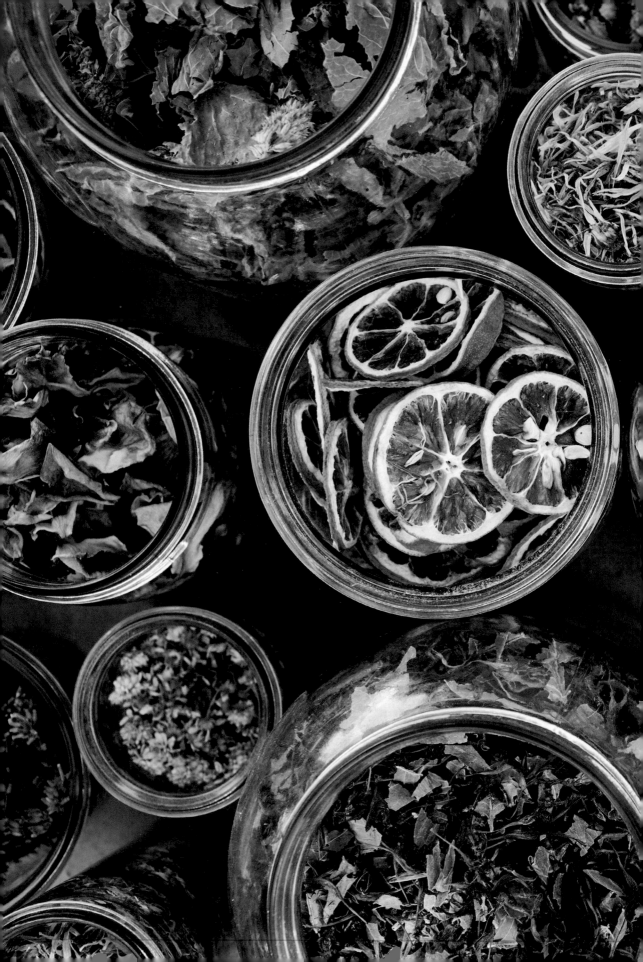

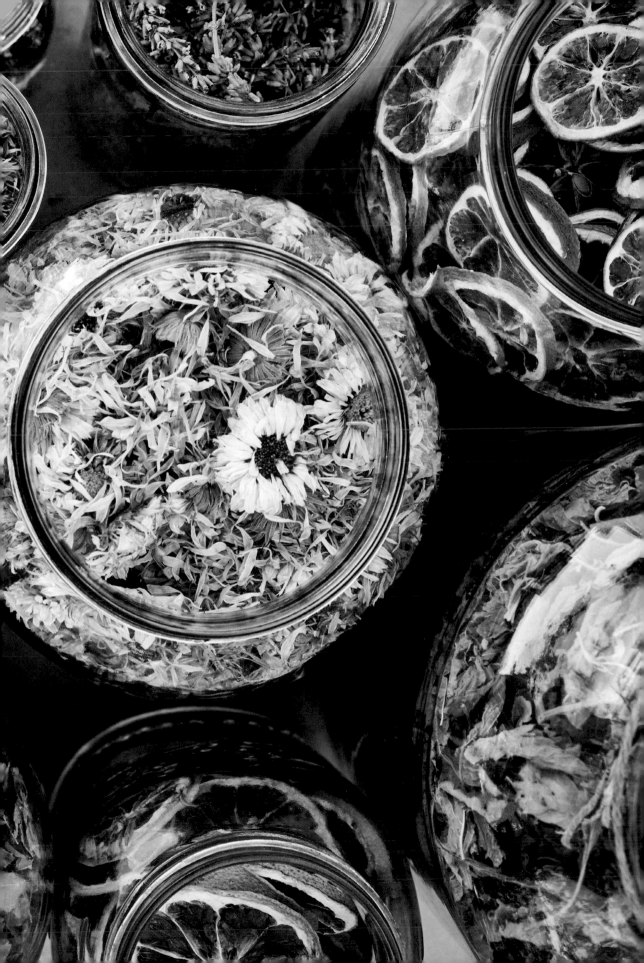

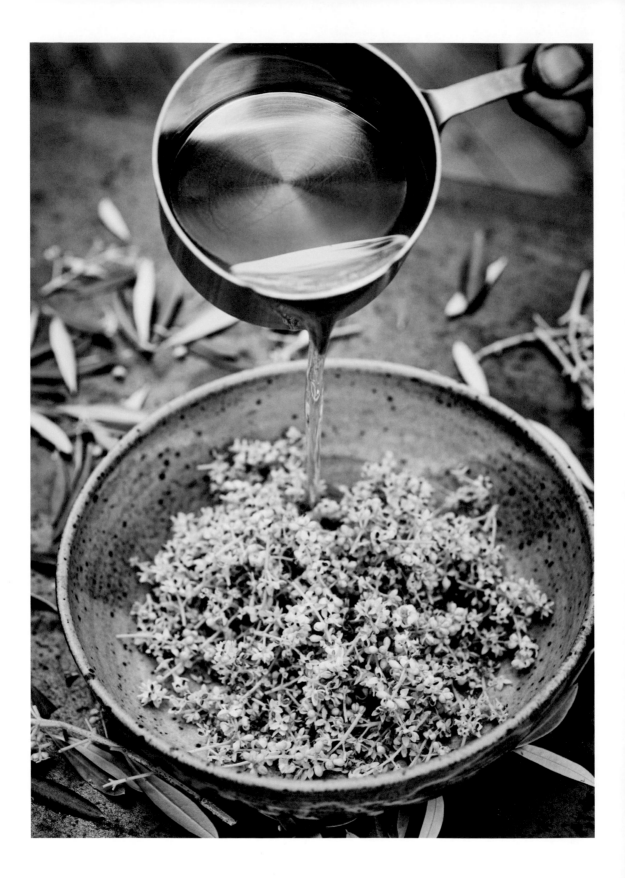

There's something magical about cultivating scents from the garden. When we are surrounded by bottles of tinctures and fragrances, jars of dried herb blends, and aromatic bushels of fresh-cut herbs awaiting the next project, we feel a bit like "kitchen witches." Alethea has always been obsessed with capturing scents. As a child, she would smash rose petals from her grandmother's rose bushes, mix them with water and spices, and sell the mixtures in front of the house. Little did she know at the time that she was already making variations of homemade fragrant beauty products.

As you spend more time using fragrant plants in your home, you can make up your own recipes and scent profiles with materials from your experiments. Many of the garden's strong, heady scents are short-lived. By capturing and preserving these scents, you can make memories of particular moments in your garden. The library of scents that you create can be used as a base for a new perfume. A blend you once used for a dry skin balm can be adjusted to create a lotion, deodorant, or pretty much anything else that you can imagine. Once you learn the basic skills of infusion, dehydration, and distillation, experiment! Keep in mind that happy accidents can occur. Sometimes a blend needs to age, and what you think smells terrible in the first hours after you make it may smell great later on.

Infusions involve transferring the fragrant parts of a plant (typically the flower or foliage, but not always) into a scentless carrier oil or alcohol medium. During the infusion process, plant parts are placed into the medium for a period of time until their scent is released, or the oil/alcohol and plants can be heated on the stove. The plant essences are transferred to the carrier oil or alcohol in this process. Dehydration removes water from plant material, preserving the plant's scent. The dried plant material can be enjoyed dried or rehydrated later in hot steam or water. Distillation captures a plant's essential oil using water vapor. Distillation creates two scented products: an essential oil and a hydrosol. Infusions and distillations can be made from a single plant source or from a blend of plants.

We take our cues from traditional perfumery techniques and keep each plant's scent profile or fragrance family in mind when blending two or more fragrant plants. As discussed on page 149, most scents consist of three combined notes: a top note, a middle or heart note, and a base note. When mixing a fragrance, you'll want to capture each of these notes.

Here are a few examples of each note from the garden:

Floral or citrus top note

FLORAL

Jasmine

Lilacs

Lilies

Roses

Tuberoses

CITRUS

Citrus

Lemon-Scented Pelargoniums

Lemon Thyme

Lemon Verbena

Spicy or herbaceous middle or heart note

SPICY

Almond Verbena

Bay Laurel

Marigolds

Pinks

Sage

HERBACEOUS

Flowering Basils

Lavender

Mint

Scented Geraniums

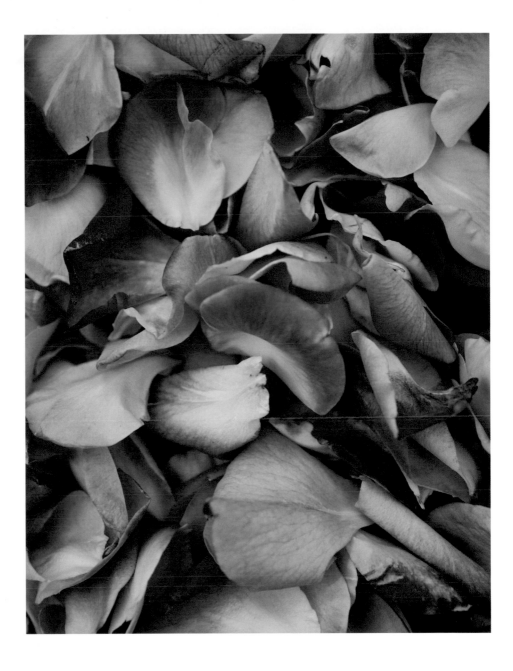

Woody base note

| Cedar, patchouli, some iris varieties

We hope you'll enjoy experimenting with different scents from your garden in the projects that follow, including a relaxing tub soak, an elegant gardenia perfume, and a heavenly lily cream. You can create wonderful treats for yourself or coveted gifts for family and friends.

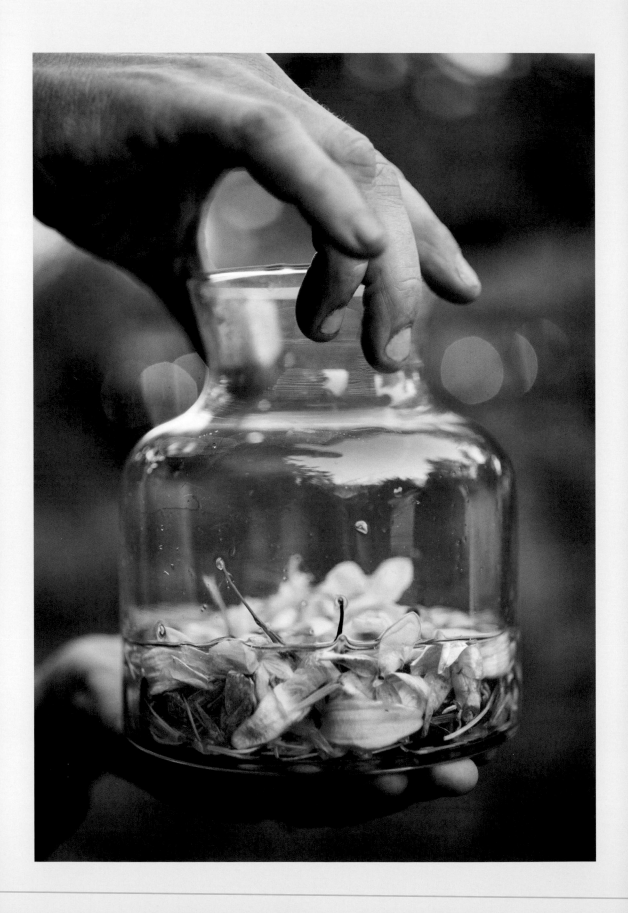

JASMINE & CITRUS BLOOMING OIL

MAKES 1 PINT

½ cup jasmine flowers
½ cup citrus flowers
2 cups jojoba oil

We blend jasmine and citrus to create a classic garden fragrance infusion to use as the basis for a nurturing scented oil. Our hardworking hands are perpetually dry and sore after hours in the garden, and we needed a hand moisturizer that hydrated our skin and stayed put through all our daily handwashings. This general-purpose oil softens and soothes tired hands, and, honestly, you can use it all over your body. Use it as a wonderful pre-shower hair mask or on dry hair to tame frizzy ends and add shine. After a shower, use it as body oil; your skin will soak it up. Use it on your cuticles, rough heels, leathery elbows—your entire body will benefit from this amazing smelling, super easy to make jasmine and citrus blooming oil.

This project can be easily doubled or halved according to how many flowers you have available in the garden. It is also a wonderful project that uses many of the fragrant plants we have shared in this book, including jasmine, honeysuckle, tuberose, gardenia, rose, citrus blossom, olive blossom, and flowering basil.

Harvest jasmine and citrus blooms when their scent is strongest, usually in midmorning to midafternoon. The flowers cannot be wet, so don't wash off any dirt or a lingering insect—brush it off instead. If flowers are harvested in the morning and are damp, allow them to dry on a cloth before beginning this infusion. It's OK if the flowers become wilted as they dry. Avoid harvesting spent flowers, instead choosing flowers that are a third to halfway open, with no signs of decay.

Fill a pint jar halfway with fresh jasmine and citrus flowers. Top off the jar with the jojoba oil, covering the flowers. Place a lid on the jar and store it in a cool, dark place for at least one week and no longer than three weeks. The length of time the flowers infuse into the oil determines how strong the fragrance will be.

After a week has passed, check the infusion, and if you like the fragrance, go ahead to the next step. If you're looking for a stronger scent, give the oil a vigorous swirl and allow the flowers to infuse for up to two more weeks, checking and swirling the oil occasionally.

When the infusion is to your liking, strain the oil into a second jar. Press or squeeze the flower heads and petals against the strainer to release the remaining infused oil. Seal the jar with a lid and store the infusion in a cool, dark place. It should keep for up to a year.

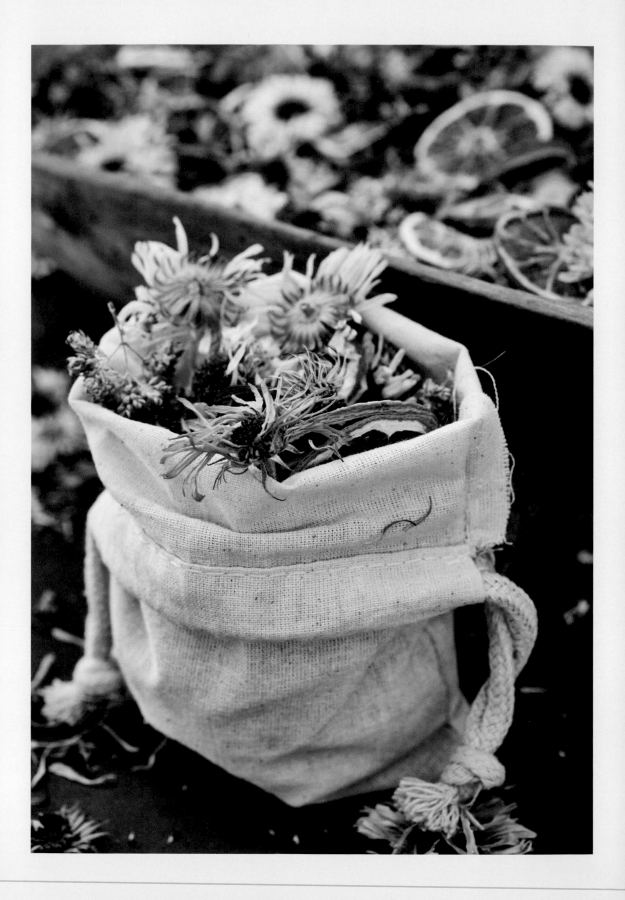

POTPOURRI TUB SOAK

MAKES ABOUT 2½ CUPS

½ to 1 cup thinly sliced citrus fruit

1 to 1½ cups fresh flowers or herbs, such as the following:

- Calendula flowers and/or petals (skin healing)
- Chamomile flowers (anti-anxiety)
- Mint leaves (antibacterial, anti-inflammatory)
- Lavender flowers (antiseptic, anti-inflammatory)
- Lemon balm leaves (calming effect)
- Oregano leaves and flowers (antibacterial)
- Snapdragon flowers (anti-inflammatory)
- Sweet osmanthus flowers (aromatherapy)
- Rose petals (anti-anxiety)

5 muslin bags, 5 by 7 inches or smaller

¼ cup Epsom salts (optional)

¼ cup dehydrated coconut milk (optional)

The potpourri tub soak is a throwback to the potpourri blends we grew up with, and we love fragrant baths! As kids of the 1970s and '80s, we remember the scented potpourris with dried fruits, leaves, and flowers in pretty little wooden bowls that were used to add fragrance to our homes. These blends were often heavily scented with essential oils or synthetic perfumes that sometimes didn't even match the scent of the dried plant material used in the potpourri! You can do better. Making your own garden-grown potpourri is not difficult and it can be used as the basis for a beautifully fragrant bath.

Drying plants is one of the oldest and easiest fragrant preserving methods. The key to maintaining fragrance in this process is to dehydrate the plants (herbs, flowers, and citrus) when they are at their most fragrant, and then store the dried plant material in an airtight container, out of direct sunlight, in a cool, dark place. When fresh plants are dried, they maintain their fragrance, although a bit muted. Once the potpourri tub soak mixture is rehydrated, the citrus, flowers, and herbs release their fragrance into the heat of the tub, with essential oils that create a restorative effect on sore muscles.

Harvest herbs, flowers, and citrus when they are at their peaks—not when plants are spent or fruits are overripe. The plant material should not be light brown or decayed. Herb foliage should be green and fresh, and flower

CONTINUED

heads should be half open or just barely open. Citrus should be firm to the touch and not overripe. If a citrus is overripe or the fruit is very mature on the stem, it will show signs of mold or will be squishy to the touch.

Gather whatever herbs, citrus, and flowers you have on hand in the garden. Oregano and calendula provide a good base with citrus for this potpourri, and you can add any other fragrant plants. It's up to you! Potpourri mixes can include calendula, osmanthus, and snapdragon. Summer blends are wonderful with rose and lavender. Once you have gathered the fresh ingredients, you're ready to start drying them.

Air-drying herbs and flowers: Bundle harvested herbs and flowers with a rubber band or a piece of natural twine. Hang the bundles upside down in a space with good air circulation and away from direct sunlight. The plants will dry in about two weeks. When they are dry to the touch and crumble easily, the drying process is complete. If the herbs or flowers are still pliable and bend easily, continue to let the plants dry.

Oven-drying citrus: Thinly slice the fruit, and lay the slices in a single layer on a parchment-lined baking sheet. Place it in a 200°F oven for five or six hours until dry.

Dehydrator-drying herbs, flowers, or citrus: A dehydrator is a fantastic tool for preserving herbs, flowers, and citrus because you can control the drying temperature and air circulation. Dehydrators are easy to use and typically come with instructions and drying times.

After you have dried the herbs, flowers, and citrus, you should have about ½ cup of dried citrus slices and 1½ cups of dried herbs and flowers. Combine the herbs, flowers, and dried citrus in a shallow bowl and mix by hand or with a wooden spoon. Transfer the mixture to a sealed jar until ready to use. The jar can be stored in a cool place out of direct sunlight for up to a year.

When you are ready to use the potpourri in a bath, spoon about a fifth of the dried blend into a muslin bag. We like to use muslin bags that are 5 by 7 inches, which have room for dried citrus, but a smaller bag also works—simply break the dried citrus slices in half, if needed, to fit into the bag.

Optionally, to elevate the bathing experience, divide the Epsom salts and dehydrated coconut milk evenly among the five bags.

Add a bag to a hot bath and enjoy!

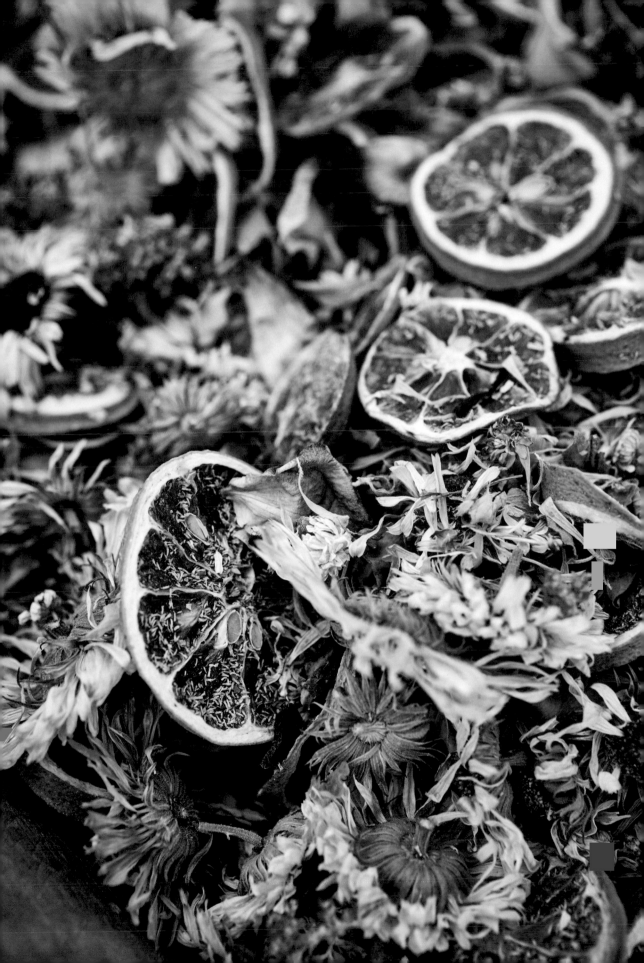

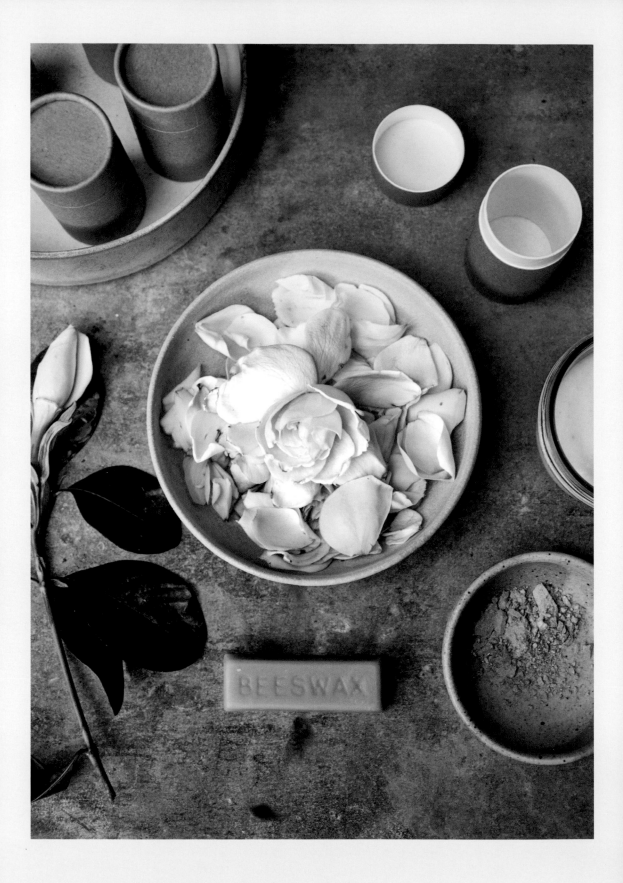

GARDENIA STICK PERFUME

MAKES 4 (0.5-OUNCE) STICKS OR
6 OR 7 (0.3-OUNCE) STICKS

2 cups gardenia flowers and petals

2 cups coconut oil, fractionated or solid

2 (1-ounce) beeswax bars

Eyeshadow or highlighter (optional)

4 push-up (0.5-ounce) paper tube containers or 6 or 7 (0.3-ounce) paper tube containers

Stick perfumes are a fun way to scent your body and take good care of your skin at the same time. Unlike flower tinctures or perfumes, you can use stick perfumes to cover yourself in scent while also hydrating your skin.

When making this stick perfume, play around with how much plant material you add to the carrier oil. If you are scent-sensitive, you can make a mildly fragrant stick by using fewer flowers. If you're a scent junkie like we are, you can heavily scent the mix by adding more flowers.

We use coconut oil in our gardenia stick perfume, but any unscented carrier oil, such as jojoba oil, will work. Infused oils can be used on their own for massage or for soothing dry skin. When you add beeswax to the scented oil, it solidifies when the mixture cools and becomes the basis for solid perfumes, salves, and lip balms.

You can add a little shimmer to this special gardenia stick perfume. The next time you break an eye shadow or makeup highlighter, don't throw it away; keep it to use to add a little sparkle to your perfume stick. If you are not growing gardenias, don't fret. You can use many fragrant flowers for this project, including lavender, roses, lilacs, mock orange, tuberoses, and more.

You can infuse gardenia flowers into an essential coconut oil in two ways: a slow method and a fast method. If you have the time, allow the flower petals to infuse their scent into the oil over a couple of weeks.

SLOW METHOD

Fill a 1-pint jar halfway with gardenia flowers and petals. Press the flowers into the jar, making sure that they are compressed. You'll need 1½ to 2 cups of compressed petals. Top off the jar with fractionated coconut oil, covering the flowers. Place a lid on the jar and store it in a cool, dark place for two or three weeks. Once every two or three days, give the jar a vigorous shake to help with the infusion process.

CONTINUED

FAST METHOD

Applying low heat can speed up the infusing process. Place either solid or fractionated coconut oil in a saucepan or small pot on the stove at the lowest heat setting. If the coconut oil is solid, stir it until it melts. After the oil has melted, add the gardenia flowers. Stir the plant material so that all parts are covered by the liquefied coconut oil. Keep the mixture at the lowest temperature, stirring occasionally. In three to eight hours, the flowers will impart their scent into the oil. The intensity of the fragrance will depend on how much plant material is used, the flowers' fragrance strength, and how fragrant you want the mixture to be.

Once the oil is infused using either method, strain it from the jar or pot into another small pot or saucepan. Press or squeeze the flowers against the strainer to release the remaining infused oil. Because the flowers will have absorbed some of the oil, there will be less oil than when you started.

Place the infusion in a pot on the stove at the lowest heat setting. Add the beeswax bars and stir until the wax melts. Once the mixture is completely liquefied, remove it from the heat.

Next, add a bit of (optional) glimmer with a neutral-colored eye shadow or some highlighter and stir. The amount you use is up to you and how much you want to shine!

Prepare the paper tubes. Use a funnel to transfer the mixture from the pot into the tubes, leaving a ¼ inch of head space at the top of each tube. If the mixture starts to solidify in the pot, return it briefly to the stove. The perfumed oil infusion and beeswax will solidify in the tube containers.

Keep a small amount of the infused liquid in the pot to top off any tubes that may develop surface cracks while drying. If this happens, simply add a little bit more of the infusion to top off the tube and allow it to cool and solidify fully.

Once the infusion is solid, place the lids on the containers and use your solid perfume frequently! The perfume lasts about six months, but odds are you will run out much earlier.

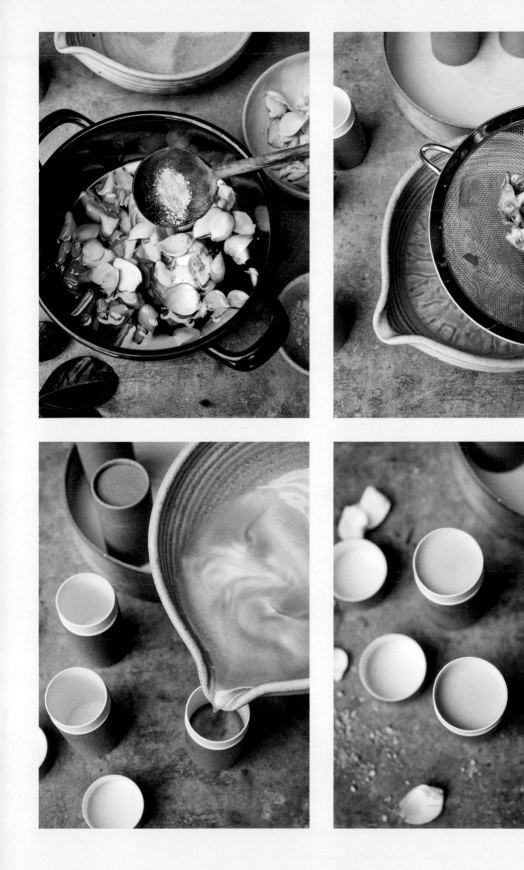

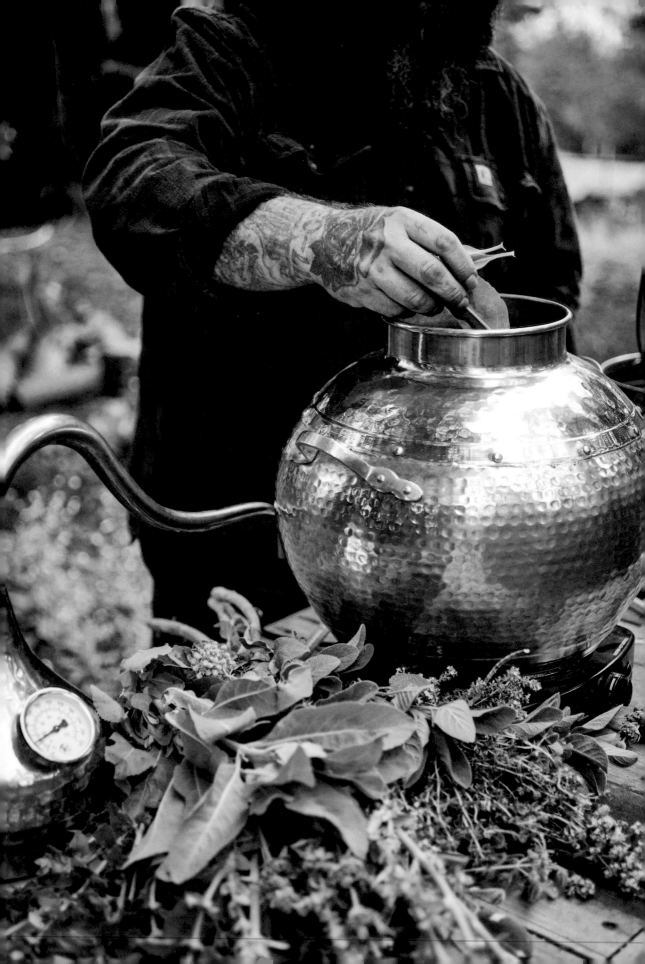

HEALING HYDROSOL

MAKES 3 OUNCES

4–6 cups fresh, fragrant plant leaves and flowers, such as white sage, oregano, Cleveland sage, and culinary thyme

3 cups distilled water

About 12 ice cubes

Hydrosols, also known as flower waters, are the water-based fragrances collected through steam distillation of plant material. The hydrosol contains the water used in the distillation process, small amounts of essential oil, and plant compounds that are extracted from your harvest. Distilling fragrant flowers and foliage is a wonderful way to preserve your garden's scents. You can use a hydrosol as a light perfume, a cooling face and body mist, the base for a facial toner, a room freshener, and so much more. We love to mix many of the medicinal garden plants we grow in our garden to make a cleansing, healing hydrosol.

Hydrosols are far less concentrated than pure essential oils, but we suggest that you start with a little, rather than a lot, with skin applications, especially if you have sensitive skin. Test a small area first with the distillation to make sure that you do not experience irritation. If you are allergic to a plant's essential oil in the garden—for example, if you get a rash when you prune a plant in the garden—you may have a reaction to that plant's hydrosol. Take note of how your body responds to fragrant plants in the garden before distilling them.

If you are serious about preserving natural scents, you might decide to purchase a still for the steam-distillation process. If you want to make hydrosols from the garden on a regular basis, a still will make this a lot easier. And if you have large quantities of a particular fragrant plant, a still will enable you to collect essential oil in the distilling process. Most stills include instructions for their use. We typically use a copper still because it disperses heat evenly throughout the apparatus and distilling equipment.

CONTINUED

If you're not quite ready to invest in a copper still, you can distill plant fragrances in your kitchen using a tall pot and lid, distilled water, and two heatproof bowls.

Once you learn the basics of distilling plants' fragrant essences, you'll have a whole new world of natural scent–making to explore! You can start with small batch hydrosols from a single plant or jump right into garden blends! All the fragrant plants shared in this book are prospective ingredients.

Harvest fragrant plants from the garden. Bring the plants indoors and gently dip them in a bowl of cold tap water to remove any unwanted dirt and insects. Place the plants on a dry cloth. Then remove foliage and flowers from stems and discard the stems.

Place a medium-sized heatproof bowl upside down in the bottom of a large pot. Scatter the plant material around the inverted bowl.

Pour the distilled water over the plant material, and then place a second heatproof bowl on top of the first, right-side up. Cover the pot with the lid placed upside down so that the knob of the lid is inside the pot.

Use medium heat to bring the water to a gentle simmer. When condensation forms on the underside of the lid, place a few ice cubes directly on top of the inverted lid or on a dish towel on top of the lid; this helps attract the plant essence–filled condensation to the center of the lid inside the pot, so that it can drip into the bowl.

Continue simmering the plant material until all of the condensed water has been collected in the top bowl. This will take about 45 minutes. Be careful to not boil longer than this, because the delicate essence can overcook or you can scorch the pot and the plants.

Remove the lid, and then remove the top bowl from inside the pot. Carefully pour the hot medicinal hydrosol from the bowl through a funnel into a sealable bottle or small jar. After the hydrosol cools, it is ready to use! Your medicinal flower water will keep up to three months in a cool place.

Collect any water left in the pot and strain the cooked plant leaves and flowers from the water. The water may be darker in color than the collected plant essence, but it will smell wonderful! Add it to your distillation or store it separately.

AROMATIC FLOWER TINCTURE

MAKES 1½ CUPS

1 cup fragrant plant material

1½–2 cups Everclear, vodka, or perfumer's alcohol

Used as a natural perfume or room spray, a scented tincture made from plants in your garden is a wonderful way to capture and preserve fragrant memories. If you make multiple tinctures throughout the growing season, you can create seasonal memories with different jars of garden fragrances throughout the year. Tinctures are also fantastic to experiment with by combining aromatic plant scents to make your own unique blends.

Creating this scented tincture is simple, but it requires a small amount of daily effort for fifteen to thirty days. Choose plants with fragrant flowers or foliage. Harvest flowers when they are most fragrant. If you're harvesting during the winter or after a summer rain, place the plant material on a cloth until it is dry to the touch. It's OK—and actually preferable—if leaves and flowers are dry to the point of wilting.

When making an alcohol-based natural scent, you'll need to use a high-proof ethanol such as Everclear, vodka, or perfumer's alcohol. For your first tincture, we recommend that you start with a single-ingredient alcohol infusion instead of placing all the plants you intend to infuse in a jar together at the get-go. Infuse the plants separately and then combine the individual tinctures once they reach the scent profile you desire. This gives you more control over the blending process and gives you time to get to know how the plant scents combine to make a final natural perfume. Once you discover favorite plant combinations, you can infuse them together, or not. Here are some of our favorite garden scent combinations:

Chamomile, lavender, and marigold

Eucalyptus, rosemary, sage, and bay laurel

Flowering basil, rose, and honeysuckle

'Mabel Grey' scented geranium and mint

Stock, citrus-scented geranium, and rose

CONTINUED

Fill a clean pint-sized mason jar with plant material, leaving a good inch of space at the top. If you're preserving a foliage scent, you may need to cut or tear the leaves to fit in the jar.

Fill the jar with alcohol to cover the plant material completely. Place a lid on the jar, and then store it in a cool place, away from direct sunlight.

Give the jar a swirl or two throughout the day. Keeping the jar in the kitchen or in another frequented room may help remind you to do this.

The next day, collect and harvest more fragrant plant material from the garden, making sure that it is completely dry before placing it in a second clean mason jar.

Strain the liquid from the first jar into the second plant-filled jar. Leave the previous day's plant material in the first jar and discard. If there is not enough liquid in the second jar to cover the new plant material, remove some material until it is totally covered by the liquid. Do not add more alcohol to cover the new plant material—this will prolong the scent preservation process by diluting the tincture.

Cover the jar with a lid, give the tincture a swirl, and wait twenty-four hours. Then collect and harvest more fragrant plant material from the garden, making sure that it is completely dry before placing it in a clean mason jar and repeat the process.

We typically continue adding and replacing small amounts of the fragrant plant material for fifteen to thirty days, until the tincture reaches a desired scent. Some plants take longer than others to release their scents; you'll need to experiment to determine the timing. You'll know when to stop the process when the tincture is infused with fragrance at the strength you desire.

After you strain the liquid for the last time, use a funnel to transfer the tincture into smaller perfume bottles or small bottles with spray heads. The tincture should be stored in a cool, dark place and used within a year.

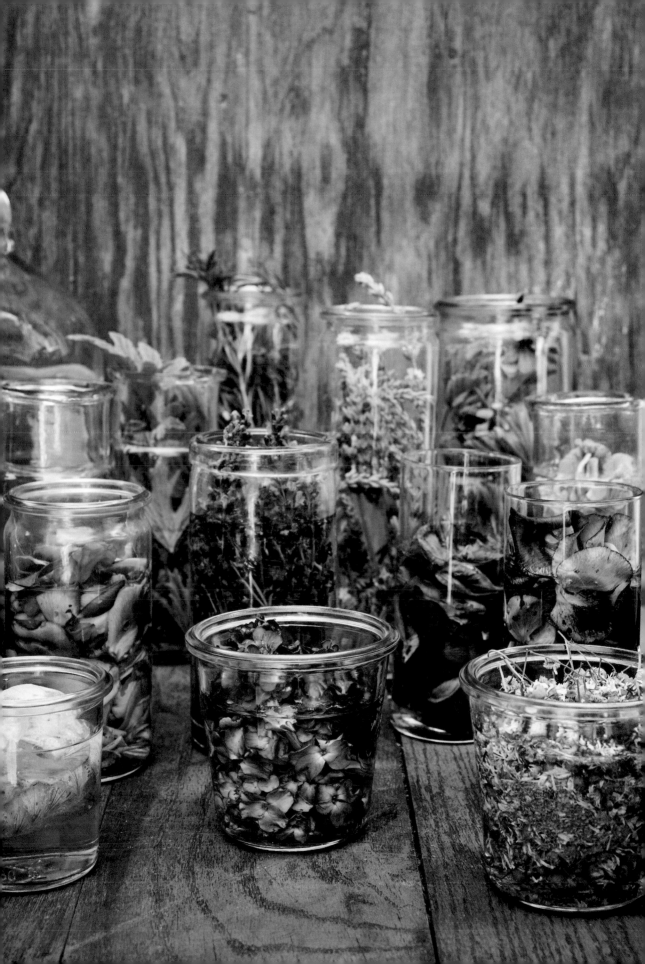

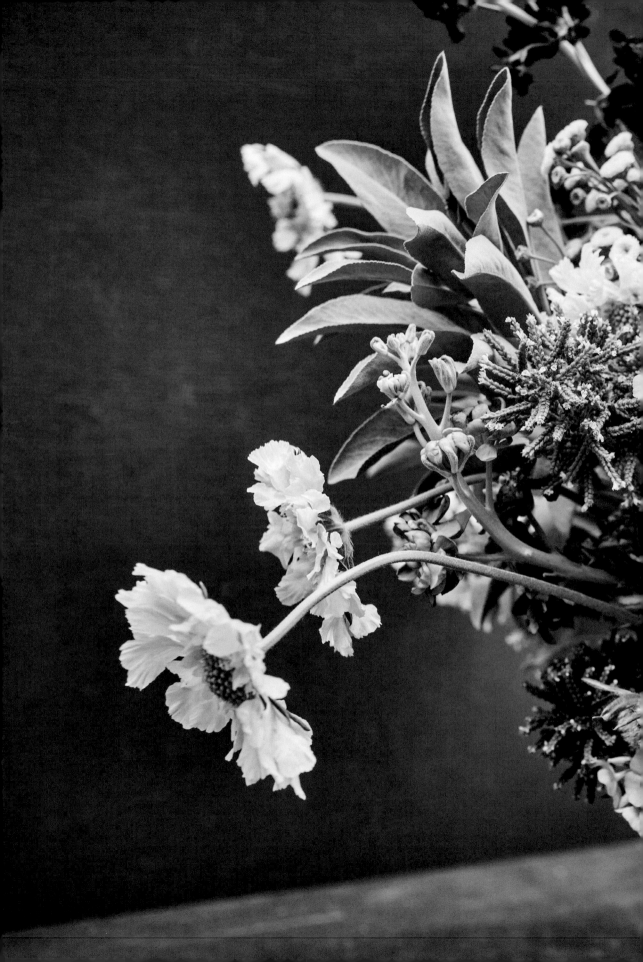

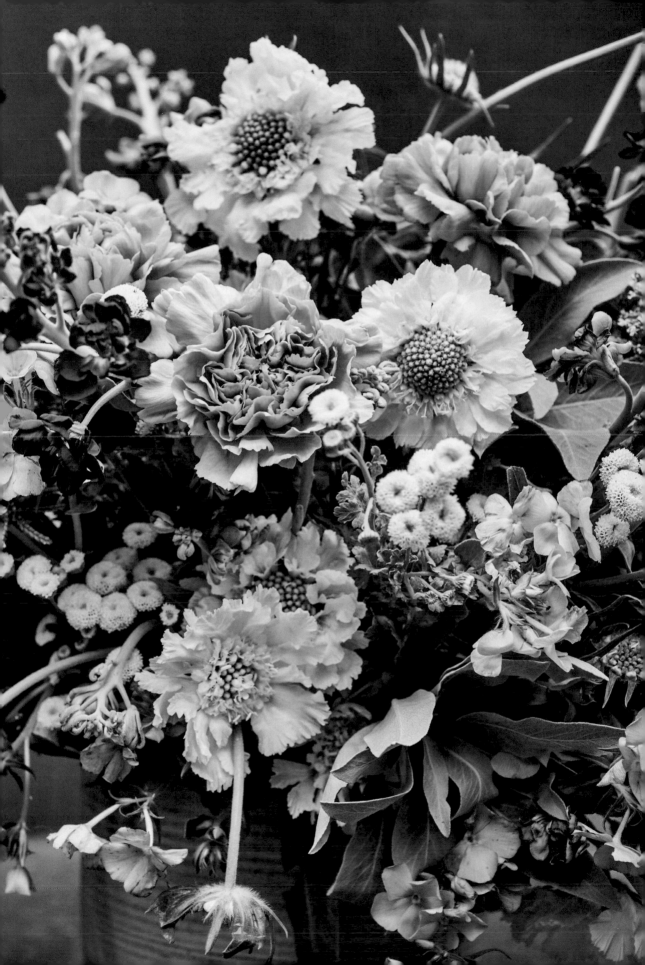

RESOURCES

Seeds

Adaptive Seeds: www.adaptiveseeds.com

Floret Flower Farm: www.floretflowers.com

Harris Seeds: www.harrisseeds.com

Johnny's Seeds: www.johnnyseeds.com

Renee's Garden Seeds: www.reneesgarden.com

Select Seeds: www.selectseeds.com

Uprising Seeds: www.uprisingorganics.com

Plant starts, rhizomes, and bulbs

Scented geraniums, flowering basils, Agastache, and herbs
Morningsun Herb Farm: www.morningsunherbfarm.com

Perennials and fragrant flowering shrubs
Digging Dog Nursery: www.diggingdog.com
Plant Delights Nursery: www.plantdelights.com

Lilies
B&D Lilies: www.bdlilies.com

Roses
Heirloom Roses: www.heirloomroses.com
David Austin Roses: www.davidaustinroses.com

Fragrant irises
Schreiner's Iris Garden: www.schreinersgardens.com

Peony, freesia, hyacinth, daffodils, and more fragrant rhizomes and bulbs
Easy to Grow Bulbs: www.easytogrowbulbs.com
High Country Gardens: www.highcountrygardens.com

Citrus trees

Four Winds Growers: www.fourwindsgrowers.com

Fruit and nut trees

Dave Wilson Nursery: www.davewilson.com

Peaceful Valley Farm & Garden Supply: www.groworganic.com

Trees of Antiquity: www.treesofantiquity.com

USDA plant hardiness zones

USDA Plant Hardiness Zone Map: https://planthardiness.ars
.usda.gov

Supplies

Copper stills

Candles & Supplies: www.candlesandsupplies.com

Push-up paper tubes

The Paper Tube Co.: www.papertube.co

Carrier oils, beeswax, and muslin bags

Mountain Rose Herbs: www.mountainroseherbs.com

Glass jars with spray tops, tins for solid perfume, and salves

SKS Bottle & Packaging: www.sks-bottle.com

Vases

Beth Katz, Mt. Washington Pottery:
www.mtwashingtonpottery.com

Beth Mullins, Studio Growsgreen Ceramics:
www.studiogrowsgreen.com

Colleen Hennessey Clayworks: www.colleenhennessey.net

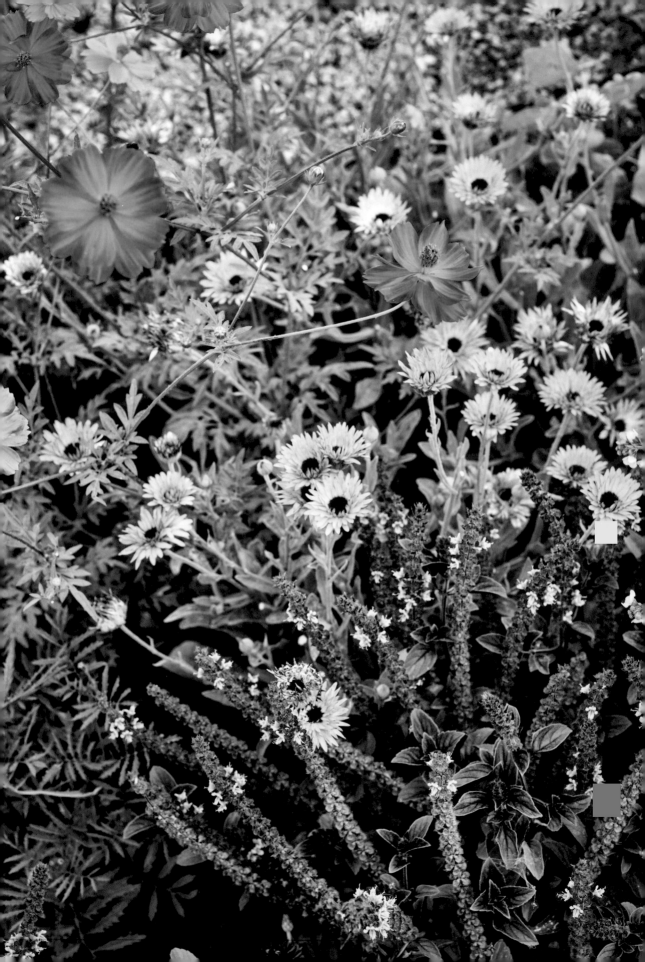

ABOUT THE CONTRIBUTORS

Stefani Bittner is the owner of Homestead Design Collective, a San Francisco Bay Area landscape design firm, and coauthor of *The Beautiful Edible Garden: Design a Stylish Outdoor Space Using Vegetables, Fruits, and Herbs*. She also coauthored *Harvest: Unexpected Projects Using 47 Extraordinary Garden Plants* with Alethea Harampolis. Stefani and her team at Homestead offer a unique and sophisticated approach, using both organic farming and fine gardening skills, for people who want help creating aesthetically designed, organic, edible gardens. Homestead provides design, installation, and full-service organic maintenance; harvesting; beekeeping; preserving; floristry; and composting services. Homestead Design Collective is the design team behind the test gardens for *Sunset* magazine. Homestead's gardens are located on commercial properties, public spaces, and private residences. Stefani and her team's work has been featured in the *San Francisco Chronicle, Wall Street Journal, Los Angeles Times, Vogue, Sunset, Food & Wine, Time, Better Homes & Gardens, Modern Farmer*, Food52, and Gardenista.com.

Alethea Harampolis is coauthor of *The Flower Recipe Book* and *The Wreath Recipe Book* and a coauthor (with Stefani Bittner) of *Harvest: Unexpected Projects Using 47 Extraordinary Garden Plants*. She is the cofounder-owner of the floral design company Studio Choo. Alethea's appreciation for the Northern California hills where she was raised, combined with a love of fine gardening, infuses her floral designs with a look that is both wild and cultivated.

David Fenton is a commercial photographer based in Oakland, California. He was the photographer for three previous books, *The Beautiful Edible Garden, Harvest*, and *The Little Bonsai Book*. To see more of his work, visit davidfenton.com.

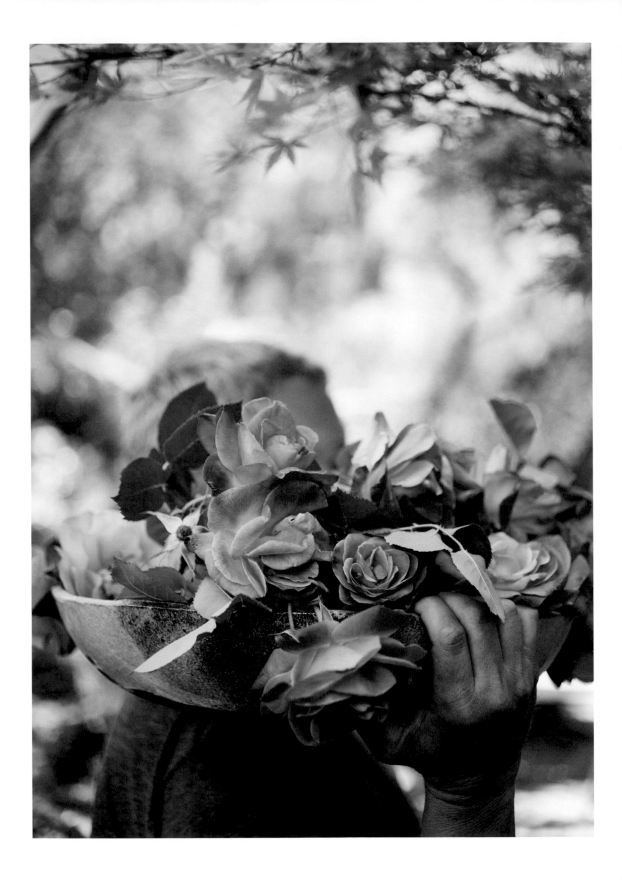

ACKNOWLEDGMENTS

We are grateful to the generous garden-loving folks in our lives who have supported and helped *The Fragrant Flower Garden* come into being. First and foremost, David Fenton, our partner in this project. Thank you, David, for your beautiful photography that captures the emotive experience of the fragrant flower garden. This book would not be the same without your skill, patience, and friendship. Thank you to our wonderful agent, Andrea Barzvi of Empire Literary, for her support and advocacy. This is our third book with the good folks at Ten Speed Press, and we have Lisa Regul, our editor, to thank for this. Thank you, Lisa for giving a gardener and florist an opportunity to write. In addition, Ten Speed's Emma Campion and Isabelle Gioffredi have lent their artistic skills to the book and Kim Keller her excellent editing skills and patience. Stefani's team at Homestead Design Collective not only created the gardens in this book but also took on the role of models in photographs of the gardens and fragrant plants. Christian Cobbs, Homestead's lead designer, shared his thoughts and experience with fragrant plants and was invaluable when we ran out of adjectives to describe scent. Peter Elliott, Homestead's project manager, also lent a hand when we were in need of additional adjectives, and he spent many hours being a soundboard for this project. Thank you to Cindy Daniels and Doug Lipton, Terry and Linda Murray, Rose Loveall, and the Flanagan family for generosity in sharing your gardens with us. Thank you to our moms, Garna and Kay, and to our daughters—who we do this for—Ana, Gil, and Ever.

INDEX

chameleon plant (*Houttuynia cordata*), 35

champak (*Magnolia champaca*), 46–47
  as anchor plant, 18
  planting ideas for, 14

Chinese wisteria (*Wisteria sinensis*), 112

chinotto orange, 40, 42

chocolate cosmos (*Cosmos atrosanguineus*),
    84–86
  in cut flower gardens, 29
  Lilies and Chocolate Cosmos, 169–70

Choisya ternata. See Mexican orange

citrus shrubs and trees (*Citrus* spp.), 41–42
  in container gardens, 34
  as focal point/destination, 17
  Jasmine and Citrus Blooming Oil, 189
  Potpourri Tub Soak, 191–92

clary sage (*Salvia sclarea*)
  A Rose Celebration, 165–68

Cleveland sage (*Salvia clevelandii*), 72
  Healing Hydrosol, 199–200
  Lilies and Chocolate Cosmos, 169–70
  planting ideas for, 14

Coleonema pulchellum. See breath of heaven

conditioning, 150

confetti bush. *See* breath of heaven

container gardens, 34

Convallaria majalis. See lily of the valley

cosmos (*Cosmos bipinnatus*)
  Lafayette Summer, 160–63

C. atrosanguineus. See chocolate cosmos

culinary gardens, 33

cut flower gardens, 23–24, 29–31

cutting tools, 151

Cyprus ironwort (*Sideritis cypria*), 100–101, 103
  as ground cover, 20
  planting ideas for, 14

D

daffodil (*Narcissus* spp.), 124, 125
  in container gardens, 34
  in cut flower gardens, 31

Daphne odora. See winter daphne

Datura spp. *See* thorn-apple

dehydration, 185

destinations, 17

Dianthus spp. *See* carnation; pinks;
    sweet William

distillation, 185

E

eucalyptus (*Eucalyptus* spp.), 43

Euphorbia spp. *See* spurge

F

feverfew (*Tanacetum parthenium*),
    102, 103–4
  in culinary and medicinal gardens, 33
  Working Herb Wreath, 172–74

flowering tobacco (*Nicotiana* spp.), 135
  in cut flower gardens, 29, 31
  Lafayette Summer, 160–63
  as night-blooming plant, 19

focal points, 17

four o'clock (*Mirabilis jalapa*), 29, 30,
    31, 134

frangipani (*Plumeria* spp.), 49
  in container gardens, 34
  as focal point/destination, 17

freesia (*Freesia* spp.), 117–18
  in container gardens, 34
  in cut flower gardens, 30, 31

fruit trees, 44. *See also* citrus shrubs
    and trees

soil, 10
Spring Explosion, 157–58
spurge (*Euphorbia* spp.), 35
Stachys spp. *See* lamb's ears
star jasmine (*Trachelospermum jasminoides*),
    19,109, 110
Stephanotis floribunda. *See* Madagascar jasmine
stinking hellebore (*Helleborus foetidus*), 35
stock (*Matthiola incana*), 132, 133
    in culinary and medicinal gardens, 33
    in cut flower gardens, 29, 31
    Spring Explosion, 157–58
sun, 11
sweet almond verbena (*Aloysia virgata*),
    14–15, 50–51
sweet alyssum (*Lobularia maritima*), 33, 130–31
sweet box (*Sarcococca* spp.), 14, 73
sweet osmanthus (*Osmanthus fragrans*), 63
    as anchor plant, 18
    planting ideas for, 14
    Potpourri Tub Soak, 191–92
    Winter Whites, 177–78
sweet pea (*Lathyrus odoratus*), 128–29
    in cut flower gardens, 29, 30, 31
    Spring Explosion, 157–58
sweet violet (*Viola odorata*), 33, 105
sweet William (*Dianthus* spp.), 86
    Lilies and Chocolate Cosmos, 169–70
sweet woodruff (*Galium odoratum*), 20
Syringa vulgaris. *See* lilac

T

Tagetes spp. *See* marigold
Tanacetum parthenium. *See* feverfew
thorn-apple (*Datura* spp.), 52
thyme (*Thymus* spp.), 104–5
    as ground cover, 20
    Healing Hydrosol, 199–200

Tincture, Aromatic Flower, 201–2
Trachelospermum jasminoides. *See* star jasmine
trillium (*Trillium* spp.), 35
Tropaeolum spp. *See* nasturtium
tuberose (*Agave amica*), 115–16
    in cut flower gardens, 31
    Winter Whites, 177–78
Tub Soak, Potpourri, 191–92
Tulbaghia spp. *See* society garlic
tulsi. *See* holy basil

V

Viburnum carlesii. *See* Korean spice viburnum
Viola odorata. *See* sweet violet

W

water, 11
white mignonette (*Reseda alba*), 31, 141–42
white sage (*Salvia apiana*), 96, 97, 99
    Healing Hydrosol, 199–200
    planting ideas for, 14
wild bergamot (*Monarda fistulosa*), 82, 83
winter daphne (*Daphne odora*), 14, 57–58, 59
winter jasmine (*Jasminum nudiflorum*), 110
Winter Whites, 177–78
wisteria (*Wisteria* spp.), 112–14
    as anchor plant, 18
    as night-blooming plant, 19
Working Herb Wreath, 172–74

Y

yarrow (*Achillea millefolium*), 29, 30, 76–77

Z

Zaluzianskya capensis. *See* night phlox

Published in the United States by Ten Speed Press, an imprint of the Crown
Publishing Group, a division of Penguin Random House LLC, New York.
TenSpeed.com

Ten Speed Press and the Ten Speed Press colophon are registered trademarks
of Penguin Random House LLC.

Typefaces: David Jonathan Ross's Roslindale and Dinamo's ABC Arizona

Library of Congress Cataloging-in-Publication Data

Names: Bittner, Stefani, 1969- author. | Harampolis, Alethea, author.
    | Fenton, David (Photographer) photographer.
Title: The fragrant flower garden : growing, arranging & preserving natural
    scents / Stefani Bittner & Alethea Harampolis ; photographs by David Fenton.
Description: California ; New York : Ten Speed Press, 2024. | Includes index.
Identifiers: LCCN 2023012424 (print) | LCCN 2023012425 (ebook)
    | ISBN 9781984860101 (hardcover) | ISBN 9781984860118 (ebook)
Subjects: LCSH: Flower gardening. | Aromatic plants. | Flowers—Odor.
    | Handbooks and manuals.
Classification: LCC SB422 .B58 2024 (print) | LCC SB422 (ebook) | DDC
    635.9/312—dc23/eng/20230825
LC record available at https://lccn.loc.gov/2023012424
LC ebook record available at https://lccn.loc.gov/2023012425

Trade Paperback ISBN: 978-1-9848-6010-1
eBook ISBN: 978-1-9848-6011-8

Printed in China

Acquiring editor: Lisa Regul | Project editor: Kim Keller
Production editor: Natalie Blachere
Designer: Isabelle Gioffredi | Art director: Emma Campion
Production designer: Mari Gill
Production manager: Dan Myers | Prepress color manager: Jane Chinn
Copyeditor: Lisa Theobald | Proofreaders: Karen Ninnis and Sasha Tropp
Indexer: Ken DellaPenta
Publicist: Lauren Chung | Marketer: Allison Renzulli

10 9 8 7 6 5 4 3 2 1

First Edition